How to Learn the Alexander Technique

Also by Barbara Conable:

What Every Musician Needs to Know about the Body

The Structures and Movement of Breathing

Also available:

What Every Pianist Needs to Know about the Body
by Thomas Mark
with supplemental material for organists by Roberta Gary and Thom Miles

How to Learn the Alexander Technique

A Manual for Students

Third Edition
Revised and Enlarged

Barbara Conable

William Conable

Andover Press
Portland, Oregon

Also distributed by:
GIA Publications, Inc.
Chicago

G-6517

Andover Press
4427 North Willis Blvd.
Portland, OR 97203

This book is published by Andover Press in Portland, Oregon, and is
available from Andover Press, www.bodymap.org. It is also distributed by
GIA Publications, Inc., Chicago, www.giamusic.com, in agreement with
Andover Press.

Also distributed by:
GIA Publications, Inc.
7404 S. Mason Ave.
Chicago, IL 60638

Illustrations adapted from *The Body Moveable*, by David Gorman, with
permission of the author.
Photographs on p. 10 by Alma Frank; used by permission of Deborah Caplan

Printed in the United States of America

5 4 3 2

ISBN 0-9622595-4-3

in memory of

Adam Alexander Conable

Table of Contents

Table of Illustrations

Preface to the 1992 Revision

Writing a book is like having a new baby. One needs to get acquainted with what one has given birth to. I produced this Manual, and I have had a little more than a year to find out what it's good for. It has more than fulfilled my hope that it would be useful to my students. My students who really live with the book and play with it, who re-read it, draw in it, write questions in it, and bring it to lessons do in fact learn faster and seem secure in their learning. Many other Alexander teachers have told me that this is so with their students as well. The Manual has been helpful to residence course students and to people who have bought it at conventions.

A use I did not anticipate for the Manual when I wrote it is for students of Alexander literate music teachers in their studios. This turns out to be an arena in which the book is enormously useful, for these music teachers know far too much about the Technique and the benefit it has been to themselves to keep it a secret from their students. But the studio teachers haven't known how to share with their students even the most basic understandings that Alexander generates. It turns out that when music students read this Manual and assimilate the ideas in it they are much better music students even when they do not have the privilege of Alexander lessons. I did not expect that. I wrote the book for persons having regular Alexander lessons, but I am not going to argue with evident success. The book does help music students who are in the studio of a body-literate teacher. The upshot is that I have made this revision very much with those teachers and students in mind.

Students' experience with the Manual has more than confirmed my belief that body mapping as developed by William Conable is an essential aid in learning the Technique. I had meant in my writing to treat the two matters of the Technique and body mapping separately, so I had intended to write a book with Bill Conable on body mapping for Alexander teachers and other teachers. Experience with the Manual has changed my mind about that. I believe we can include in this book all that is essential in the mapping work and keep it in the hands of the people who need it most, our students.

Another motive for this decision is the ringing in my inner ears of a line from the Stephen Mitchell translation of the *Tao Te Ching*, "In thinking, keep to the simple." Body mapping shares with the Alexander Technique the supreme virtue of elegant simplicity. I find that when the idea of body mapping is presented simply and straight-forwardly people will expand and elaborate it according to their needs. A singer needs an accurate and detailed map of breathing, a potter does not, but the potter had better understand wrists really well. Both singer and potter need a profound comprehension of primary control, which each recovers more easily in the context of an increasingly detailed and accurate body map.

Preface to the Third Edition

The biggest change in this edition is incorporating into earlier chapters all the information of relevance to everyone from the chapters that were formerly addressed to actors, dancers, and musicians. Material specific to actors, dancers, and musicians remains in their chapters, and those chapters are now appendices. I made this change because I learned that most people who are not actors, dancers, or musicians do not read those chapters no matter how relevant the information contained in the chapters might be, for instance, about breathing! I'm hoping this change will make all the information more available to everyone.

Beyond that, I have reworked almost every page of the book, reflecting both my learning and the advice and feedback I have had about the book from others. In the earlier editions I made an appeal for suggestions for changes that would make the book increasingly useful for students and teachers of the Technique. Many people responded, some with a sentence or two, and some with many pages of analysis and constructive criticism. I am very grateful for this gracious help, and I have used it, even when I have perhaps seemed not to. Some people wanted me to put a lot more about inhibition in the book on the understanding that inhibition is so central to the Technique that a book without it can't be about the Technique. I agree that inhibition is a crucial component of constructive conscious control and the concept of inhibition and its practice informs every page of this book, even the body mapping sections: one cannot institute an accurate map without suspending the old inaccurate one. The concept of inhibition and the practice are here. I have attempted to make that even more explicit in this edition.

I have watched people use this book to transform themselves and their experience. How is this book well used? Suppose you buy the book in July of 1995. How might it look in July of 1997 when it goes on the permanent shelf along with assimilated dream journals, diaries, and vacation photographs? Tattered. Riffled. Underlined. Highlighted in several colors. Full of notes, questions and answers. Full of Mind Maps and drawings. Full of quotes from other books about the Technique and pictures stapled in or paper-clipped. It might look comfortably and happily lived in like your home, and your body. I wish you comfortable and happy learning.

I am writing now in September of 2004, on the occasion of my distribution agreement with GIA Publications, Inc. in Chicago. I enter into this agreement with joy and gratitude, chiefly because I hold the folks at GIA in such very high regard, and I am thrilled to be associated with them in a new way. Our agreement will result, I have no doubt, in people finding this book who might not otherwise have found it. This pleases me because over the years I have been told so many wonderful stories about the benefits that come from the book. A woman told me that the UPS man, when he delivered her copy, told her excitedly that he wouldn't be working if a friend hadn't given him this book. He had suffered from back pain as he delivered boxes, to the point of almost quitting. When he learned from this book how to move properly and sit properly in his job, he was free of pain.

It is deeply gratifying to learn how much the book has helped people. May the benefits to you, new reader, be very great as well.

— Barbara Conable

I. Welcome to the Study of the Alexander Technique

This workbook is designed to aid you in your study of the Technique. Keep it near you, work in it daily or as often as you like, browse in it, play with it, enjoy it.

> The Alexander Technique is a simple and practical method for improving ease and freedom of movement, balance, support, flexibility, and coordination. It enhances performance and is therefore a valued tool for actors, dancers, and musicians. Practice of the Technique refines and heightens kinesthetic sensitivity, offering the performer a control which is fluid and lively rather than rigid. It provides a means whereby the use of a part—a voice or an arm or a leg—is improved by improving the use of the whole body.

These are Alexander's principles, or Alexander's discoveries, as some call them:

> *Primary Control*
>
> Primary control is the inherent and intrinsic mechanism for balance and support in the body. It assures that uprightness will be effortless and that movement will be supported and fluid. Primary control depends, as we shall see, on the preservation or the recovery of a dynamic relationship between the head and the spine in movement or in stillness.

> ### Downward Pull
>
> If we are meant to be effortlessly upright, why do so many of us experience effort in being upright? Because we interfere with the intrinsic sources of balance and support. We impose a pattern of tension throughout the body that compromises the primary control. Alexander called that pattern of tension downward pull.

> ### Constructive Conscious Control
>
> Alexander learned that it is possible to consciously inhibit the imposed pattern of tension he called downward pull and to consciously cooperate with and facilitate the primary control and thereby recover grace and poise in movement and ease in sitting or standing.

(You may be thinking as many other students have that this is an odd use of the word *control*. If so, perhaps it will help you as it did me to consult a dictionary. I found several definitions of control that emphasize domination or command, but then I found one definition of control as guidance or regulation. I believe it is constructive conscious guidance or regulation that Alexander had in mind, a conscious cooperating with the fountain of psychomotor support within.)

I formulate Alexander's discoveries as Laws of Human Movement, laws in the scientific sense, universal and invariable. I believe there are two.

> I. Habituated tensing of the muscles of the neck results in a predictable and inevitable tensing of the whole body. Release out of the tensing in the whole must begin with release in the muscles in the neck.
>
> II. In movement, when it's free, the head leads and the body follows. More particularly, the head leads and the spine follows in sequence.

The next few pages examine these Laws, so that you may understand exactly how they work.

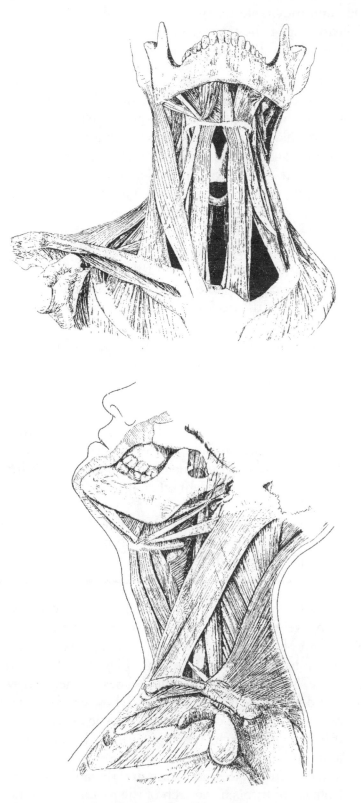

The Muscles of the Neck

Law of Human Movement I: Habitual tensing of the muscles of the neck results in a predictable and inevitable tensing of the whole body. Release out of the tensing in the whole begins with release in the muscles in the neck.

The muscles on the previous page are the most important muscle group in the body in the matter of freedom and ease of movement. If you tense the neck muscles as you move you will experience a consequent tensing of your whole body. No other muscle group has that power. If you tense other muscle groups—abdominals or buttocks muscles for instance—there will be local accommodation to that tensing which will be idiosyncratic, particular to you and to the circumstance. But if you tense neck muscles, you will suffer a contraction that will be global in your body and that will look and feel very much the same in you as it does in other people. It is this contracting of the whole body in response to the habitual contracting of the muscles of the neck that is called downward pull.

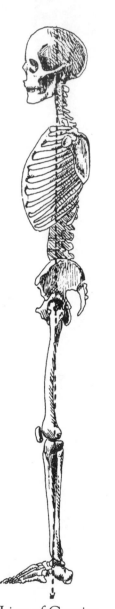

Line of Gravity

Why does the condition of the muscles of the neck determine the condition of the whole in movement? For two reasons:

> 1. Tensing in the neck distorts the rest relationship of bone to bone in the skeletal system, impairing the skeleton's ability to deliver weight efficiently.
>
> 2. Tensing in the neck interferes with involuntary muscular support for voluntary movement.

Reason number one can be readily understood by examining weight delivery in the skeleton. Notice that the weight of the head centers on the weight-bearing part of the spine, which is its front half. (The back half of the spine, looked at from the side, houses the nervous system and does not bear weight.) Notice how weight is delivered down through the cervical and thoracic curves of the spine into the large weight-bearing vertebrae between the ribs and the pelvis. Then the weight passes into the hip joint and on through the knee joint and the ankle joint and from there through the arch of the foot and into the ground. This is beautiful and efficient architecture.

That is, the architecture is efficient until or unless we tighten the muscles of our neck, in which case the efficiency is compromised. Because the muscles of the neck are head-moving muscles and because a tightened muscle shortens, when we tighten the muscles of our neck the head is pulled off its rest relationship with the spine and a series of compensations ensues. Typically, the upper spine drops backward, putting pressure on the lower back. To relieve the pressure on the lower back the pelvis will most often tilt in a way that pulls the hip joints forward, and then the legs tighten and ease at the knee and ankle is lost. This results in an alteration in the gait as well as an effort in uprightness. The rest relationship of the arm structure to the spine is also distorted in ways that we will examine in detail later on. It is the whole body contraction described in this paragraph that we call *downward pull*.

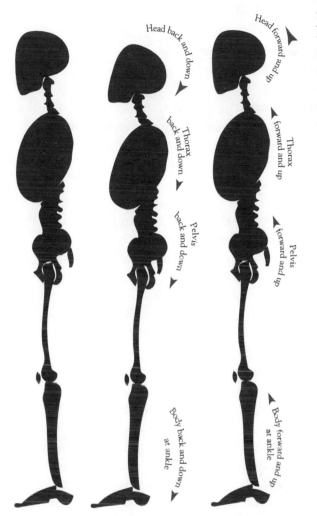

Balance   Downward Pull   Back to Balance

The whole contracting pattern begins with the alteration of the relationship of the head with the spine, because the shortening neck muscles move the head and their contraction becomes habitual. The head does not get to return to the rest relationship. That distortion is disastrous for the quality of head movement, for the rest relationship is that place from which movement in any direction is easiest. In fact, the mobility of the head will be restricted to the degree that muscles tighten.

How does the head-spine relationship change when neck muscles tighten? The head is pulled 1) forward of the spine, and 2) closer to the floor, and at the same time 3) it tilts backward.

Alexander named two of these three directions when he said the head moves down and back in misuse. He named down toward the floor (2), and he named the tilting backward (3). He did not name (1), the dragging of the head as a whole *forward* of the spine. It is important to name the forward dimension of this movement, because students who know that their head must move forward and up in order to recover the rest relationship with the spine will sometimes feel the head as a whole moving back in relation to the spine and feel that they are doing something wrong. No, they are simply noticing the movement of the head in relation to the spine rather than the movement of the head forward out of its backward tilt. Got it?

To recapitulate: reason number one why the condition of the neck muscles determines the condition of the whole is because their habitual tightening distorts our skeleton in a way that prevents its delivering weight efficiently. It is compensation for the loss of that efficiency that we feel as effort in uprightness.

Reason number two why the condition of the neck muscles determines the condition of the whole is that the postural support for the body is compromised by downward pull. This compromising of support was first researched definitively by Frank Pierce Jones at Tufts University. You may read about that research in his book (*see the bibliography*) and in his numerous articles in medical and scientific journals, soon to be published together by Richard Brown. Other scientists are duplicating Jones' work and carrying on to a complete understanding of postural mechanisms in the body. This manual will not attempt to even summarize the scientific information on this matter because it is so readily available to you elsewhere and because it is the practical application of what is verified in that work that concerns us here.

What is of profound practical importance is this. There are two categories of muscular activity, voluntary and involuntary. Voluntary activity we experience directly. When I move my arm to reach for a glass of water I know that I am moving it and I feel the sensation of its moving overtly, as movement. But I can feel only indirectly the involuntary muscular activity that keeps me upright as I reach for the glass, just as I can feel only indirectly the beating of my heart or the rise and fall of my diaphragm. Rather, I feel involuntary work indirectly, as a sense of being supported or balanced or heart-beated or breathed. If humans felt involuntary work directly as we do the moving of an arm we would be overwhelmed with sensation.

But here's the rub. The pattern of tensing Alexander called downward pull interferes with or opposes or counters the involuntary patterns that support us. Typically those involuntary patterns lengthen us, especially when they involve the spine. Downward pull shortens us. The result is effort in being upright which many people come to accept as normal, confusing the effort of compensation with the effort of uprightness. People are so accustomed to effort that when they get their first taste of effortless uprightness since childhood they sometimes feel like they will fall.

Worse, voluntary movement loses quality to the degree that it loses its involuntary support. Suppose I reach for a glass of water. If I am allowing the free flow of my postural responses to the movement I will feel balanced and supported and my reaching for the glass will feel easy and buoyant. If not, I will feel the background effort *and* an inordinate effort in reaching for the glass.

So, we might state the purpose of the Alexander Technique in one sentence: The purpose of the Alexander Technique is to learn to take optimal advantage of the bony structure (mechanical advantage, in Alexander's words) and of involuntary muscular support for voluntary movement.

> **Law of Human Movement II: In movement when it's free the head leads and the body follows. More particularly, the head leads and the spine follows in sequence.**

The head leading–spine following pattern is common to all vertebrates, so it can be observed in nature wherever you go. I find that people often have readiest access to what they already know about the head leading if they think of animal movement. Do you remember what a cat does when it gets up from resting? The first thing that happens is that its head begins to move at the location of the head's joint with the spine. (Remember that we only move at joints, so if a head is to move, it must move at its joint, its joint with the spine.) Then there is a wave of activation down the cat's spine that lasts half a second. There is a perceptible lengthening of the spine as this activation occurs. The cat's back seems to come to life. It is only then that the cat's legs become involved. The limbs seem to fit in naturally in their turn with the lively moving that has activated the spine. Then wherever the cat goes—up on a sofa, down off a sofa, dipping its head to a bowl to drink, tumbling with another cat, around a corner, even backing up—the head leads the spine, and that *primary movement* (Alexander's first name for the primary control) continues as the context in which all other movement occurs. If you can imagine the cat's movement clearly you have a handle on the primary movement the Alexander Technique can liberate in you.

Now remember where you have seen the same thing in human movement. You have, no doubt, seen the primary movement in action in some fine athletes, dancers, and musicians. These persons activate in vertical motion the same reflexive support for movement that the cat activates horizontally. The very same. And that support, that lengthening, gives human movement the same grace and wholeness we admire in animals.

Or watch a baby crawl. I love it when my students bring a baby to a lesson. Then we can watch the baby and see her little head lead and her body follow, and we can crawl with the baby. A week before this writing I taught at

Memphis State and had the good fortune that a baby of about ten months came to class with her mother. The baby was in a cheerful mood and eager to move and soon she was in the middle of the studio with twenty dancers around her imitating every move she made. She thought this was very amusing and she gave the dancers lots to imitate. That baby taught those young dancers more about the sources of grace and freedom in the body than I could have taught them without her in many hours. Her primary control was not imprisoned by counter-contraction.

I watched the dancers learn from that baby a greater trust of their own bodies. I watched them figure out that the same organization and support the baby had was intrinsic to them and could be liberated. They learned that they could consciously cooperate with that involuntary pattern, that they could consciously experience that pattern as a potent impulse toward lengthening in their spines. Later in the session they discovered that if they rode that impulse as they went up on toe or bent their knees they got a movement that was buoyant and organized and led easily into the next movement.

Sometimes people are frustrated in liberating their primary control by a discouraging sense of the power of habit, the strength of the downward pull. I tell them, "Be frustrated, but don't be discouraged, because no matter how powerful habit is, it doesn't begin to compare to the power of the primary control. Primary control takes two thousand pound polar bears over ten-foot cliffs as if they weighed nothing. I saw it myself at the St. Louis zoo. No matter how old your habits of contraction are, they are not as old as your primary control, which you have had since a few weeks after your conception. And the miraculous thing is that primary control is never impaired, even by decades of counter-contraction. It waits there in your spine like a bulb in winter waiting for the sun of your intelligence to shine on it so that it can bloom." A. R. Alexander once said, "Be patient, stick to principle, and it will all open up like a great cauliflower."

Pitfall

Think of any adventure story that comes to mind and you will remember how many dangers the hero or heroine encountered and overcame, how many sloughs or temptations or dragons or evils, on the way to the prize. Your adventure in liberating your primary control has only one major pitfall besides the discouragement I have already mentioned and that is a trying to DO it, rather than to free it. If instead of allowing the lengthening of your spine you try to lengthen your spine with voluntary movement of the sort that picks up glasses of water you will not get what you are after but something quite different: not a freeing, but a stiffening; not a lengthening, but a stretching sensation; not buoyancy, but boundness; not support, but struggle; not freedom, but posture (yuck). If you find yourself doing that, give it up. Go to the zoo, or eat some ice cream, or read a mystery, and come back to the whole matter again later and re-think it.

There *is* doing in re-learning primary control, but it is doing of a subtle and sophisticated sort. It the doing of cooperation. You voluntarily, 100 percent on-purpose cooperate with that intrinsic, inherent vital support. So there is also non-doing. The pattern you are cooperating with you could not possibly *do* any more than you can beat your own heart. It is built into you at the deepest level physiologically. I am reminded of Psalm 139. My primary control has been with me since "thou didst knit me together in my mother's womb." Our task is to restore the original stitches. Our goal is a second innocence.

To illustrate this further I have included on the next pages a picture of F. M. Alexander after he recovered the grace of his primary control. Notice the ease in his body, the effortlessness of his uprightness. Then observe the same thing in the child. The child's is a first innocence, Alexander's a second.

The saving word in avoiding the pitfall of doing is intention. If your intention is freedom, if your intention is restoring natural spinal organization and support, if your intention is strong and clear, you will succeed. The power of your intention will carry you past any tendency to overdo. My *American College Dictionary* defines intention as the "act of determining mentally upon some action or result." If you are determining mentally upon freedom and support, you will succeed.

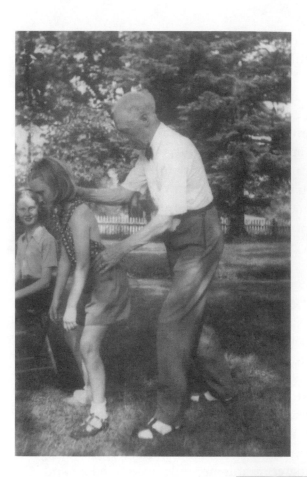

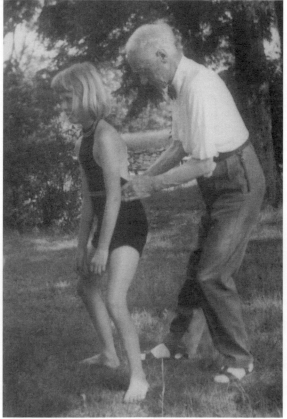

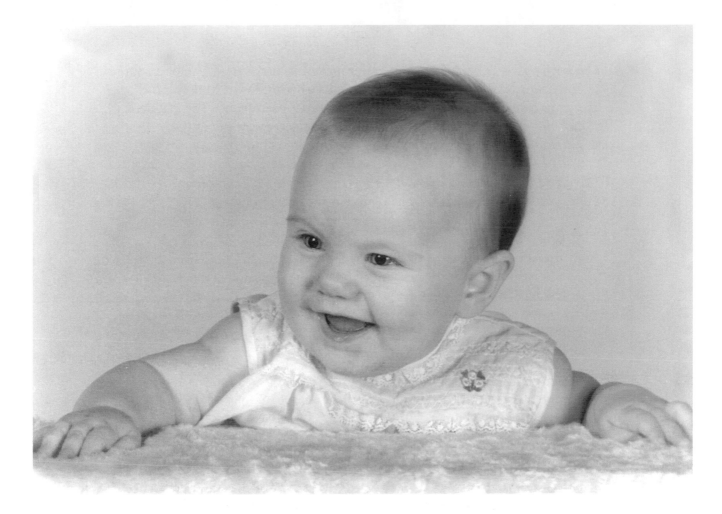

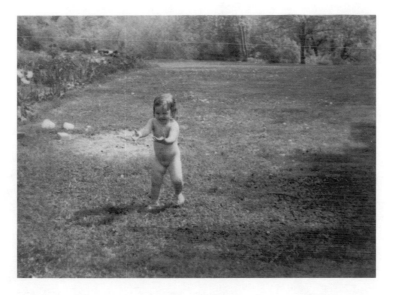

F. M. Alexander's Books

If you wish to read about how Alexander made his discoveries, the best source is his own words. Alexander wrote four books which Edward Maisel has edited into a single paperback called *The Alexander Technique: The Essential Writings of F. M. Alexander*. I recommend this selected reading over the longer original volumes for most purposes.

To give you the flavor of Alexander's writing, here is a paragraph of his on the primary control from his book *The Universal Constant in Living*:

> When I was experimenting with various ways of using myself in the attempt to improve the functioning of my vocal organs, I discovered that a certain use of the head in relation to the neck, and of the head and neck in relation to the torso and the other parts of the organism, if consciously and continuously employed, ensures, as was shown in my case, the establishment of a manner of use of the self *as a whole* which provides the best conditions for raising the standard of the functioning of the various mechanisms, organs, and systems. I found that in practice this use of the parts, beginning with the use of the head in relation to the neck, constituted a primary control of the mechanisms *as a whole*, involving control *in process* right through the organism, and that when I interfered with the employment of the primary control of my manner of use, this was always associated with a lowering of the standard of my general functioning. This brought me to realize that I had found a way by which we can judge whether the influence of our manner of use is affecting our general functioning adversely or otherwise, the criterion being whether or not this manner of use is interfering with the correct employment of the primary control.

II. Downward Pull

Downward pull is the pattern of tension in the whole body that originates with habitual tension in the neck. The eyes accommodate the chronic backward drag of the head by shifting in the orbit and they are chronically partially lidded. The jaw loses mobility and juts forward in opening. The tongue bunches and the throat tightens. The vertebrae of the neck are jammed together, putting pressure on nerves and blood vessels, creating a susceptibility to tension headaches. Breathing is impaired, vital capacity decreased, rib mobility decreased; the movement of breathing becomes disorganized. The spine loses range as well as its ability to lengthen and sequence in movement. Pressure is put on internal organs. The arm structure is distorted. The shoulder blades are pulled together as the back narrows and there is also a caving-in of the chest, dragging the collarbones down and in; in other words, we narrow front and back. The upper arm is torqued outward, rotation is compromised at the elbow, there is retraction across the wrist, and the hands tense. Meanwhile the whole back shortens and narrows. The lumbar area is shortened and forced forward, or back. The gluteals shorten, forcing the hip joints forward in space. The pelvic floor is tightened uncomfortably upward. The thighs torque outward, putting pressure on the knees and causing the muscles of the lower leg to tighten, hardening the area between the tibia and the fibula. The lower leg is pulled off the perpendicular at the arch, forcing weight onto the heel, or, in extreme cases, onto the ball of the foot. The foot torques, the heel pulling to the inside and the front of the foot twisting outward, often sufficiently so that the reflexes that give us a sense of a spring in the step are lost. Toes lose mobility.

Students justifiably inquire, "Why do we pull down?" I tell them I have heard downward pull ascribed to varying sources, among them imitation of parents or teachers, fearfulness, attempting to reduce sensation or emotion, a reaction to pain, a sense of worthlessness or defeat, a mechanism for staying where one doesn't want to be, a means to prevent violence, a means of feeling smaller. Frank Jones believed that downward pull is habituated startle; Thomas Hanna seems to concur (see his *Somatics*.) Others believe it is caused by premature uprightness in infancy.

Now ethologists, anthropologists and others have become interested in dominance and submission and their physiological and gestural indicators, such as dipping the head, hunching the shoulders, and dropping the eyes. It may be that humans habituate submissive posturing.

This question of the cause(s) of downward pull is very important. Someone is going to answer it definitively some day. It might be you.

III. The Laws of the Spine

> I. THE HEAD MUST LEAD.
>
> II. THE VERTEBRAE MUST FOLLOW IN SEQUENCE.
>
> III. THE SPINE MUST LENGTHEN IN MOVEMENT.
>
> IV. THE MOVEMENT SHOULD BE EQUALLY DISTRIBUTED AMONG THE JOINTS OF THE SPINE.

I. The Head Must Lead

One might think of the head as a highly elaborated top vertebra, made larger by nature in order to accommodate the brain and the eyes and ears and speech and facial expression. There are many millions of years of evolution behind leading with the head, even pre-vertebrate evolution. Bill Conable once gave an introductory lecture about the Alexander Technique in which he said, "How *can* you tell which is the front end of a worm, anyway?" Ever since creatures extended roundness into longness, heads have been leading bodies. Raymond Dart, the great anatomist, said: "All invertebrates, from the segmented worm and caterpillar to the crustacean and insect, and all vertebrates, from fish to man, are built on the same sort of linear plan" (*The Attainment of Poise*). Learn to watch every sort of creature with this central dynamic of the body in mind. When the head is leading and the spine following, all movement is organized and supported dynamically, and it is that organization and support that gives movement breathtaking beauty and integrity.

Sometimes people imagine that the head should lead from the top of the head. No, that's not where it leads from, and people who try to lead from the top of the head always stiffen instead of free. The head leads from the joint of the head with the top vertebra, the occiput with the atlas, to use the fancier names. That's the joint at which the head moves in any case. This case of the head leading the spine into length and into movement is no different.

II. The Vertebrae Must Follow in Sequence.

Sequencing throughout the spine cannot occur if the head doesn't lead. You can verify that right where you sit. Suppose you want to bend your torso over your lap. If your head leads and your spine is not frozen by tension in some part of it you will experience a sequencing down your spine. If your spine is frozen in some places you can still experience the sequencing, it will just skip over the frozen part. Now repeat the movement and do not allow your head to lead. Notice that you are obligated to initiate somewhere else, probably in your lower back, and the movement is a scattered chaos, resulting in a shortening of the spine.

In either case, after you bent over your lap you were obligated to unbend to order to be upright again. In the case of unbending, your head initiates your spine's lengthening and the sequencing in the vertebrae is from the bottom of the spine to the top. If you didn't understand that last sentence just reread it and experiment until you get it. I don't know how to say it any more clearly. Or watch the sequencing. All little children unbend that way. The little head goes on forward and up in relation to the spine so that the whole spine lengthens, which allows the little child to unbend vertebra by vertebra from the bottom to the top. Cats do the same as they put their paws up on the furniture. Their heads initiate the half-second lengthening of their spines which allows a successful initiation of the spinal movement from the tail to the head that gets the cats paws onto the coffee table.

It's a wonderful thing to watch a dancer unbend whose spinal sequencing bottom to top is secured by the lively lengthening of her whole spine. Without the primary movement from the top of the spine to the bottom, the secondary movement from the bottom to the top is chaotic and often ugly.

III. The Spine Must Lengthen

The spine either lengthens in movement or it shortens. Don't take my word for it. Watch and watch. Experiment. Inquire. Mess around. This insight is worth anything it takes to understand it.

IV. The Bent Spine Should Distribute Movement Equally among the Joints

Sirens go off in the spine when this law is disobeyed. The spinal police write lots of tickets for this one. Suppose you are reading a book at a desk and you have your head and neck bent forward so that most of the bending is concentrated just at the place where the cervical curve gives way to the thoracic. Your trapezius muscle will burn, you will be very stiff when you finish reading, your neck will be tighter, and you will have reduced mobility at your joint of your head with your spine. If, on the other hand, you distribute the movement evenly across the vertebrae you get an easy curving of the whole torso over the desk and you feel fine. I call this desk yoga. It's good for you.

IV. Learning the Alexander Technique: A Model

This simple model has helped my students gauge their progress in learning. If we imagine a continuum with the left end representing the tensest a person could be and the right, the freest,

tense   free

←——————————————————————————————→

then we can understand that no one comes to the Technique at one point on the continuum but rather within a range on it, so that the student will be tenser sometimes and freer other times.

tense   range   free

←—————————(——————)——————————————→

The student will have some ability to negotiate the range, some strategies for freeing. As the student learns, the range will shift and, presumably, widen.

tense   free

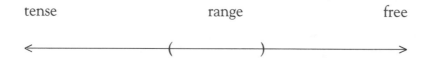

←————(————{————)————}————→

The student will notice that some tensing falls away forever. The student might report, "I used to always tighten my whole upper torso and meet the oboe half way when I brought it up to play. Now I never do that. I just bring the oboe to me." That old tensing would fall on the continuum between (and {. At the same time, the student reports new freedom, "And last night I sat through all of George's bassoon recital and I didn't have any of the aching and burning across my shoulders that I usually have at bassoon concerts." That new freedom would fall on the continuum between) and }.

The model is a reassuring one. It saves the misery of the Am I There Yet? question by crediting a range of experience, and it focuses attention on strategies for reliably negotiating the student's current range on the continuum. It promotes an ideal of gradual experimentation and liberation rather than of Getting There.

The model reassures in another way which for some students is critically important. It allows for a continual progress from left to right of { } without the necessity of moving (. This gives the student permission to choose all his old behaviors if he needs them, or when he needs them. Such a student might end up with a range like this:

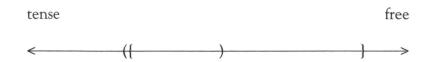

tense   free

The student who benefits by this choice is the student who attributes meaning to the old behavior that makes it very important to keep it in the repertoire. Sometimes students tell me that the old contracting feels protective. One young man said, "I love the new freedom when I'm with my friends or playing my French horn, but when I go home at Christmas time I pull right back down again in order to feel safe. I think if my dad saw me all lengthened out and easy he'd punch me out." That young man needs his downward pull for those occasions, and later he noticed on his own that to pull down on purpose is experientially different than to do it unawares. Later he may be confident enough to test his sense of danger, knowing that he can always pull back down if it turns out to be correct that ease and presence antagonize his father.

Musicians in transition from tense playing to free playing also need that permission to return to familiar strategies, especially in performance situations, until they have really assimilated the new use. I tell them to use rigid control to whatever degree they need it until they feel really confident of fluid control. Performances early in learning will often exhibit some of each, and that's fine, especially if the performer has a videotape of the performance and can watch it many times in order to see what he has done and how it has worked.

You may use the remainder of this page to create a continuum for yourself on which you may chart your own progress toward freedom. You will be providing your brain with visual feedback to augment the kinesthetic feedback of your increasing freedom. Brains thrive on feedback.

V. How Alexander Teachers Use Their Hands

Alexander Technique teachers *teach* with their hands. A crucial distinction must be made at the outset, the distinction between teaching and treating. You may come to your first Alexander lesson having had treatment of various sorts from the hands of persons who give treatments with their hands. You may therefore associate the use of hands with treatment in your mind, and unless you add a new category in your mind, the category of *teaching* with hands, you may be handicapped in your learning. People who give treatments with their hands are massage therapists, osteopaths, chiropractors, reiki practitioners, and the like. They all mark the same occupation box on their tax forms with the medical doctors, who also treat with their hands, as when they repair a wound with stitches. Alexander Technique teachers do not mark that occupation box on their tax forms; rather they mark the teacher box, which they share with music teachers, dance teachers, golf pros, tennis coaches, etc., all of whom sometimes teach with their hands. Like these other teachers Alexander teachers have many modes of communication available to them, talking, visual aids, imitating, modeling, mirrors, text, and teaching with their hands.

In treatment situations success or failure depends on the treater and on the appropriateness of the treatment and the skill with which it is carried out. A physician who fails in treatment is liable to suspension; but in college it is the student who fails to learn who is liable to suspension. Patients are not suspended, and teachers are not responsible for outcome in the same way surgeons are. I make the distinction this baldly because so much depends on the student's disposition. A passive student who imitates the attitude and behavior of a patient or client will not learn properly.

Students, take an active role in your learning the Technique. Imitate what Alexander did in discovering the Technique. Observe. Question. Experiment. Inhibit your old habits and wait for something more profound to emerge. Cooperate with the new as it emerges. Bring the full power of your remarkable brain to bear on your learning so that you can assimilate it into your very being, as you would a new language. Be playful with what you learn, as you would if you were taking a cooking class.

Another clue to this being a teacher-student relationship that your are entering, not a doctor-patient or a treater-client relationship, is the Code of Ethics your teacher honors. It is a teachers' code, not a treaters', and you may obtain a copy of it by writing to the American Society for the Alexander Technique, or Alexander Technique International, addresses for which are in the chapter on selecting your teachers.

VI. Your Kinesthetic Sense and How to Use It in Learning the Technique

In order to learn the Alexander Technique comfortably and easily you need to understand the sensory mode you are using as you learn. Just as you would be primarily using your visual sense if you went to the museum to take a course in painting or your auditory sense if you took a music course, so you are using a particular sense, your movement sense, as you learn Alexander's Technique. The difference is this. Your mother and father, as representatives of the culture at large, named seeing and hearing for you. They taught you directly the difference between blue and green and loud and soft. They probably did not, on the other hand, name kinesthesia for you, nor did they directly teach you basic kinesthetic distinctions like tense and free or balanced and unbalanced.

The fact is there are six senses, and we name five. In addition to sight and hearing and touch and taste and smelling we have a movement sense, known more technically as the kinesthetic sense. The kinesthetic sense tells you about your body: its position and its size and whether it's moving and, if so, where and how. That is the information that corresponds to color, depth, and shape in vision or salt, sweet, and bitter in the gustatory sense.

In order to be very clear about this, do a simple experiment. Put a hand over your head where you can't see it. Notice that you know right where the hand is, though you are not doing anything we ordinarily call sensing. Notice that you could describe in detail your hand's position. You could say how the fingers relate to each other and to the palm, where the hand is in relation to your head or to the floor, whether there is a bend at the wrist. Now wiggle your fingers. Notice how much you know about the wiggling. You could say when you started, when you stopped, the speed, the sequence, whether the palm was involved, what joints were moving. Now imagine that your little finger grew four inches. Notice that if that were to happen you would know it from the inside. You would not need to look.

Notice something else before you bring your hand down. Look at your hand and notice that you begin to use your eyes as your main source of information about your hand. That inner sense of its location fades. Now do the same experiment with your tactile sense—no longer look at your hand, but instead reach up and feel it. Notice how you begin to rely on your second hand to tell you where the first one is.

I do not know whether this preference for any other sense than our kinesthetic reflects a cultural prejudice or whether there is a built-in sensory
hierarchy. My guess is that it is the former. After all, a sense that is not even
named is unlikely to be trained. If a sense is not named or trained we do not
have the easy commerce with it that we have with senses we name and train,
like vision.

Notice some other things about your movement sense. First, notice that you
can form a gestalt of any size or complexity with your movement sense as you
can with any other. I mean *gestalt* in the old, original sense, that is, the contents of your consciousness at any moment and its organization. When you
had your hand over your head you very likely narrowed your consciousness to
only your hand. You were not including those other parts of your body, arms,
torso, and feet. You could have been wiggling your left foot or uncomfortable
in your knee and probably you would not have known it because your attention wasn't there. But notice now how complete your kinesthesia can be. Find
the hand you had over your head wherever it happens to be right now and
notice its position. Now expand your attention to take in your arm, then your
arms and torso. Include your head, and then your legs, so that all of you is in
your awareness. Now find your hand in relation to the whole of you, and
notice that you can go on noticing relations among parts within the whole in
very complex and interesting ways.

This ability to notice the part within the whole is critical to easy learning of
the Technique, because in the Technique we notice what we are doing with
our heads in their poise on the spine. We need to be able to sense how the
whole body changes when the neck frees and the head finds its balance on
the spine. We need to be able to allow adjustments back toward balance in all
the joints.

Notice also about your kinesthetic sense that its use is effortless, as is every
sense. If I ask you to notice the color of the wall nearest you, what do you do?
You simply turn your attention in that direction and effortlessly register the
color. Or if I ask you what sounds you can hear at the moment, you turn your
attention toward hearing and effortlessly notice sounds that may not have
been in your awareness at all a moment ago. Similarly, if I ask you now to find
your right foot kinesthetically, you make the same maneuver of consciousness.
You turn your attention toward your foot and there it is! effortlessly, and
instantly.

Notice also that nothing prevents your going on noticing kinesthetically just
because you happen to be seeing and hearing, too. So you can notice them all
at once, wall and sounds and foot. It isn't true that we can only do one thing
at a time. In fact, we can do many things at once. Some professions require
that an astonishing amount be happening in consciousness at once. Orchestra
conducting comes to mind. Think of the conductor! She is shaping the

movement, indicating the tempo, balancing the violins and violas, cueing the timpani, and saying to the oboe, "No, no, it's G *sharp*." At the same time she had better be awake in her body, her whole body, or the orchestra will not realize the liveliness or the feeling the music requires. This is not a matter of rapidly going from item to item in consciousness, what I call scanning. No. Scanning can be done, but it doesn't work well for activities such as conducting. Rather, consciousness seems to organize in concentric circles, item within item, with an ever-fluid focus within the whole.

So, with the Alexander Technique, if we do not already have it, we develop the ability to bring body feeling into consciousness in a comfortable, ongoing way. Most people experience this as a kind of coming home. There is a relief in it, in becoming embodied again. It turns out the effort is not in feeling our bodies but in not feeling them.

We learn to live in a kind of sensory soup. To the onions of vision and the garlic of hearing we add the carrots of kinesthesia and the potatoes of the tactile and the *fines herbes*, taste and smell. There is a richness in this that is homey and gratifying for most of us and essential for the artist. Artists with a reduced consciousness live their professional lives with a serious handicap.

How to Use Your Movement Sense in Your Alexander Work

Some Alexander teachers avoid the question, "How does that feel?" I do not avoid it because I believe that a student's experience is her very best feedback. Suppose I guide a movement in a student that reduces her downward pull and enhances her reflex support. I might ask her:

Me: How does that feel?

Student: Well, it feels better. It's a little hard to say how.

Me: Grope a little. We all have trouble describing kinesthetic things in the beginning because we weren't taught to.

Student: Well, it certainly feels lighter, and my shoulders are less tense. I almost always hurt up here across my shoulders [she rubs her hand across her upper back], but I don't now.

Me: What else do you notice?

Student: I feel taller.

Me: How much taller?

Student: Well, I feel about six inches taller.

Me: What do you suppose is the truth of it?

Student: Oh, I'm really a little taller because I was so scrunched before, but I'm not six inches taller.

Me: Yes.

Student: I also feel sort of tipped forward.

Me: What do you suppose the truth of that is?

Student: Well, I know I'm used to throwing my weight backward because I carry my head so far forward.

Me: Take a look in the mirror. [She is standing sideways to it.]

Student: Well, I'm upright. [She giggles.] In fact, it looks like I'm still a little back even though I feel like I'm forward.

Me: Why, do you suppose?

Student: Probably because I'm so used to it.

Me: Yes.

Student: I'd go back where I was so I could see it, but I'm afraid I couldn't get out of it.

Me: Go ahead. I'll help you again if necessary.

Student: [She goes back into her habit, shortening herself and throwing her weight backward to counter her head.] Gosh, that looks awful. I look dumpy.........I can't believe how far back I am............No wonder my lower back hurts. There's so much pressure on it..............And I keep trying to tuck [she tucks her pelvis] to get out of it. It helps a little but it tightens my legs. [She plays with the angle of her pelvis a little bit and makes a face and shrugs.]..........I hate it down here. [She giggles.]

Me: Explore it a minute—you've got the light of consciousness shining on your habit.

Student: [Looking away from the mirror.] I think this is shorter than I really am.

Me: Yes.

Student: Scrunching like this pulls my shoulder blades closer together.

Me: Yes.

Student: I'd like to get out of this!

Me: Go ahead.

Student: [She straightens herself. She makes a face.]

Me: How does that feel?

Student: Kind of pulled up.

Me: That's how it looks, too. What else?

Student: My shoulders hurt again and my legs are tight.

Me: How come?

Student: I don't know exactly, but I think I did something real different than I did with your guidance.

Me: In what way?

Student: Well, this was sort of forced, and when you guided me I sort of glided up.

Me: What else do you know about it?

Student: I kind of pushed from my back, but when you guided me we started with my head.

Me: Right. That makes all the difference. You're designed to move with your head leading. It's built right into you, that pattern.

Student: [Scrunching back down.] Let me try again. [She starts to push again from her mid-back.] Oops, no. That's the old thing. Hang on. [She pulls back down again, then after some thought she moves easily up with her head leading.] That's it. That's better.

Me: How do you know?

Student: Because it was easy and it feels good again.

Me: In what way?

Student: I feel taller, but not stretched.

Me: What else?

Student: Less pain in my shoulders.

Me: How come?

Student: It seems like when my head pulls forward and my upper back drops back my shoulders get caught in the middle, like two opposing forces pulling on them. [She giggles.]

Me: I'll say they do.

Student: This must be why I get so tired playing the violin.

Me: Yes. To the work of scrunching you add the work of playing. Bodies love to play the violin, but they hate to scrunch and then play. It isn't in the job description.

Student: I still feel tipped forward, though.

Me: Go forward to where you feel like you are.

Student: [She tilts forward several inches.] That's where I feel like I am. [Laughs.]

Me: Notice that you couldn't go there if you were there! Now go back to balance.

Student: [She goes past balance back toward habit.] Oops, that's too far. [She comes back to balance.] There's a lot less work going on here.

Me: Right.

Notice that the student has begun to process her own kinesthetic experience in a way that will help her. This is exactly what Alexander did in the early days of his explorations. Ms. Student makes up a kinesthetic category, scrunch, to name her experience. It's a rough equivalent of downward pull, but she knows exactly what she means, and it is sufficient for the moment. The first time I heard a symphony orchestra I called it pretty. Now I could say more sophisticated things about it, like it was Szell-ish, or baroqued-up, or out of tune. Later Ms. Student will find sophisticated kinesthetic categories, but for now scrunch is fine. It lets her examine what she does.

Notice that she begins to figure out for herself that there are ways in which her kinesthesia isn't reliable (Alexander made much in his writings of our sensory unreliability). She feels six inches taller, but she is only a little taller. She feels tipped forward when she comes to balance because she is used to tipping backward. I explain to her that this is simple sensory accommodation, like an orchestra getting used to a higher A, and that in a very short time upright will feel upright. Kinesthesia corrects very quickly when a person experiences it in context, with relevant distinctions. The sound of a minor chord is easier to identify if one had heard it in relation to a major chord in the beginning. That is why I encouraged Ms. Student to go where she felt like she was, to give her another reference point.

Notice also, and this is very important, that there are ways in which her senses are perfectly reliable. She knows perfectly well when she is lighter or freer or when something is easier or better balanced or more supported or more comfortable. I have never had a single student with any sensory unreliability in discerning these qualities, so in the beginning I encourage students to focus on those qualities as they examine their experience. Noticing kinesthetic qualities also serves as wonderful feedback for them when they are on the right track, or the wrong. I tell them, "If it's lighter, freer, easier, better balanced, more supported, more comfortable, it's it. Nothing but cooperating with primary control and our design makes us feel that way. Contracting against primary control makes us feel heavier, tenser, more effortful, unbalanced, unsupported, or uncomfortable. This is true in general and it is true in the particular."

My expectation is that Ms. Student will go on exploring in a like manner between lessons. I call it constructive messin' around, and the students learn fastest who do the most of it. I have learned to judge my teaching not by how someone is when he leaves my teaching room but by how he is when he returns. Many students make significant improvements in use between the time they leave and the time they return. Alexander said, "You can do what I do if you do what I did." The difference is that our students have the benefit of all he learned in his constructive messin' around as they do their own.

Kinesthesia Is Only One Element in Body Awareness

Body awareness is comprised of many elements. Kinesthesia is one of them, and I have emphasized it here because it functions so importantly in learning Alexander's ideas, but the other elements of body awareness are of equal importance for life and for artistic expression, so I want now to put kinesthesia in this larger, essential context.

Another element in body awareness is the *tactile sense*. Tactile sensation is, of course, in the skin. Persons vary greatly in their awareness of tactile sensation, hot and cold, pressure (as from clothing), texture. Sometimes musicians are handicapped by an over-reliance on the tactile. There are pianists, for instance, who read almost everything they do off what they call the feel of the keys. Their sense of movement in their hands is then reduced in some cases to almost nothing, so that if I ask them to raise their hands from the keyboard and make the same movements in the air that they have just made in relation to the keys, it feels very strange to them, almost ghostly, they may tell me. In that case it is very important to balance their tactile experience with kinesthesia so that they can discern the effort they are using to depress the keys, which will in these cases always be excessive. On the other hand, there are violinists who have very little tactile appreciation of the string. When I inquire into this I often find that they learned to numb out or ignore the tactile sensation of the string because as children, before they developed calluses, the string hurt their fingers. Now the numbing is a handicap to them because they lose the sensitivity to the string that makes a pleasing vibrato possible.

There are actors who are very tactile in their approach. They touch themselves in their roles in ways that enhance the role or they feel the props tactually in a way that speaks or they feel the elements. I want Lear to feel the rain and the wind on his face. When that tactility is married to kinesthesia, when skin and muscle are both awake, wonderful things happen on stage.

I find people with a highly developed tactile sense have an asset in learning Alexander's ideas even if their movement sense needs work. They have at the same time a sense of body boundary and of body contact with the world that helps them, especially if they can readily translate a tactile impression into a movement response, as when following the guidance of a teacher's hands in moving.

Other

—*Proprioception*. I had used the word proprioception in earlier versions of this book as Arnold Mindell and others do, as a sort of grab-bag term inclusive of every bodily sensation not kinesthetic or tactile. (Neurolinguistic Programming practitioners, by the way, use kinesthetic to include *all* bodily sensation.) I acknowledged that some persons use it as a term roughly equivalent to kinesthesia and that others use it with a very narrow meaning confined to certain kinds of kinesthetic sensation arising from particular kinds of receptors. More recently those other uses of the word have prevailed, and I feel obliged to change my terms. Fewer and fewer people use the word the way I did, and the advocates of the word *proprioception* are prominent. Oliver Sacks argues the point in *A Leg to Stand On:* "There used to be another old word, still often used—kinesthesia, or the sense of movement—but 'proprioception,' less euphonious, seems an altogether better word, because it implies a sense of what is 'proper'—that by which the body knows itself, and has itself as 'property.' One may be said to 'own' or 'possess' one's body—at least its limbs and movable parts—by virtue of a constant flow of incoming information, arising ceaselessly, throughout life, from the muscles, joints and tendons. One has oneself, one *is* oneself, because the body knows itself, confirms itself, at all times, by this sixth sense. I wondered how much the absurd dualism of philosophy since Descartes might have been avoided by a proper understanding of 'proprioception.'"

Now, I'm not going to be argued out of my use of the "old" word, kinesthesia, only my use of proprioception. I would always choose a more euphonious word over a less, and I'm far more enamored of the root *kin* than I am of the root *prop*. The *kin* root always signifies movement, and movement is what it's all about. I give up proprioception without a fight, but not kinesthesia.

So what do we do with all those elements of body awareness I used to subsume under the grab-bag term of proprioception? Name them all, I guess, letting them stand individually as coequals with the others, thus snatching victory out of the jaws of defeat. So:

—*Pain*. The PET scanners have proven all known theories of pain wrong, and pain experts are driven to come up with new theories compatible with the highly consistent and mysterious imaging of pain the scanners presented to the experts. Meanwhile, pain is a present and compelling reality in the lives of many Alexander Technique students. Indeed, many students come to the Technique because of pain for which there seems to be no medical remedy. In many cases the Technique is the only agency for relief available. An example is the ubiquitous back pain which most of the time is caused by misuse and cannot be relieved except by correcting the mis-use. Deborah Caplan, who is a physical therapist as well as an Alexander teacher, has written an entire book about the application of Alexander's ideas to back pain. It's called *Back Trouble*, and if you have back trouble you should read *Back Trouble*.

The teacher and the student must first determine together whether the pain is in fact use-related. If I have any doubt I recommend that a student first be checked out medically. Most of the time, in most of the complaints that come to me, doctors find nothing, or nothing treatable. In some cases, movement retraining serves as a valuable adjunct to surgery or drugs or physical therapy. In the case of numbness in the arms, a frequent complaint among musicians, I ask the student to be checked by a neurologist. In only one case of numbness has a brain tumor been detected. One is enough to justify a lifetime of caution, in my opinion.

The teacher and the student must determine whether the pain is use-related. Sometimes that it is use-related, that is, simply caused by the manner of use that the student brings to the joint or the affected area, is readily evident to the teacher. Sometimes it takes time to determine whether it is and we are only certain when we see that pain reduces in proportion as freedom increases. Other times we assume in retrospect that the pain was use-related because with lessons it disappears. This will most often be true of pain that was not even reported in the beginning, but only later, "You know, before I had lessons I had a lot of tension headaches, and now I never have them." "Oh, good."

When there is severe pain and the student has little kinesthetic sensitivity we really have our work cut out for us. I tell the student that what she must do in the beginning is like learning to listen to the flute with the trumpets blaring. It can be done, but it takes intention. The flute in this case is the kinesthetic sensations of increased lightness and ease and buoyancy, even if those qualities come in tiny increments. I can tell you that students in severe pain are not immediately impressed with initial small increases in lightness, but I ask them to continue to notice them anyway, along with any increments of reduction of pain. I tell these students they have two barometers instead of one. They can monitor the relationship between increased ease and decreased pain, both over time and in the moment. I tell them it is very important to keep refining the ease and freedom barometer because one of these days the pain barometer will be gone. The pain can function as a biofeedback, which of course it is! If you sit at the computer in a mechanically disadvantageous way the buzzer in your lower back will go off as pain. Then you must make a response to that stimulus that eliminates the pain and go on sitting at the computer in a mechanically advantageous way or the buzzer will go off again.

Often I recommend that a student be very alert and sensitive to the relationship between use and pain and to keep a careful record of it, in a notebook or a computer or a tiny tape recorder the student can carry in a pocket. If students are videotaping their activity they can voice record their experience and later they can correlate their reported comfort with what they see on the screen. There is a world of learning in this. Once a student comprehends that good use correlates with comfort and bad use with discomfort, motivation and a willingness to process experience are secure.

When students come for lessons because of discomfort I look for an important turning point in their experience, from what I call the "wolf-from-the-door" phase to the "where's-my-good-ole-buoyancy?" phase. In the beginning all the student wants is to be free of the discomfort and success is predicated on that. Later the student comes to value the kinesthetic qualities the Technique makes it possible for him to enjoy and he continues to study in order to enhance his experience.

—*Pleasure*. There are unnumbered kinds of pleasure available in the body, unnumbered varieties of sensation that may go by that name. A body in a natural state is a sea of pleasure, even in grievous circumstances. Pleasure is reduced by downward pull, as is all feeling, and the recovering of the natural bodily pleasures is a good indicator of success in the application of the Technique. Added to myriad pleasures that are not kinesthetic is often a growing delight in movement. Just as one may take pleasure in seeing, or take pleasure in hearing, so one may take pleasure in moving. The primary control itself is distinctly pleasurable. One of my dancer students reported to me recently that dancing had become truly joyous for her. I wasn't surprised.

—*Micromotion*. This phenomenon is definitely a component of body awareness and it is certainly related to pleasure in the sense that it is pleasurable. One may delight in it. A free body feels like a body in motion even when it is in positions we usually categorize as still, like sitting and standing and lying down. Micromotion is all the sensation of the activity going on in the body. It must be complex, to say the least. It must include the muscular activity that keeps us reflexively upright (a sort of kinesthetic hum), the flow of fluids, the subtler sensations of breathing. Micromovement feels small-scale, too, almost as if we can feel activity in cells. There's no proof we can feel activity in cells, but if we could it might feel like what I am describing. I never mention micromotion to my students until they experience it on their own. They say, "I feel like a willow in the wind," or, "I'm standing still but I feel like I'm dancing!" or, "I feel like I'm standing on a body." This is an appropriate use of metaphor. Freedom seems to turn people into poets spontaneously.

—*Emotion*. Emotion, whatever else it is, is sensation. When a wave of fear or anger or joy sweeps over us we experience it at least to some degree as a wave of sensation. Students differ in their interpretation of that sensation, especially in the relationship they believe it has to their tensing. Some say that tensing is an expression of their emotion, others that it is a resistance to it. "I tense because I don't want to feel the fear that I have." Or the anger.

Sometimes a release into freedom or an unfamiliar movement is accompanied by a wave of emotion. A student might say, "I suddenly feel so sad." More and more students are accomplished at processing emotion as it arises; they accept emotion; they express it appropriately or report it. Some students are in therapy at the same time that they are studying the Technique and if they are lucky they have in the therapist a resource for integrating the emotional and the physical. Many therapists, however, do not know much about the Technique, and Alexander teachers are not trained to deal with emotional issues. This limitation on both sides will, I believe, over the next few generations be removed. More therapists are seeing the benefits of body work for their clients as well as for themselves and more Alexander teachers are comfortable when their students express emotion in their lessons. In the case of the Alexander Technique, it used to be that if a student cried the teacher would often be disturbed or terminate the lesson. More often now the teacher will make a more supportive response and find, in fact, that the crying facilitates the process toward freedom and awareness.

If you are learning the Technique while working through serious emotional issues it may be that you will be helped by reading the chapter in this book entitled "If You Have Suffered Abuse or Violence." Sometimes emotional abuse in a person's life requires a healing process as thoroughgoing and intense as healing from physical abuse. In any case, feel free to discuss with your teacher what she can offer that will support your healing. Alexander teachers are for the most part very clear about their limitations in this regard, and their assets. There are now Alexander teachers in training as psychotherapists and some who are skilled co-counselors. Just ask.

A final word here to psychotherapists themselves. A number of therapists have come to me because they are physically uncomfortable as they work. I teach them as I would any other student who must sit for long periods of time. And I encourage them to pay special attention to the portions of this book that deal with body awareness. My students who are uncomfortable as they do therapy often report that they become almost entirely exterospective as they work. All their attention is on their client and little or none is given to themselves. This is a liability for therapists in two ways. First, it limits their information about their clients to what they receive visually or auditorily. Their own bodily responses to the clients are unavailable to them. The magnitude of this loss is only clear when compared with therapists who have those responses available to consciousness and report that they are sources of their most valuable information about the client. Secondly, the loading of awareness onto the client in preference to the therapist is a burden to the client. I tease therapists when they do that. I say, "I know it feels to you like this means I'm Really Listening, but to your client it probably feels more like I'm Just as Upset about this as You Are." Therapists who learn to maintain a unified field of attention tell me they are less tired at the end of the day. Sometimes, they say less drained!

—Hunger and thirst. Sometimes students discover how profoundly they reduce body awareness when they realize that they can go literally for hours without realizing that they are thirsty or hungry. Or that they have to go to the bathroom. When you recover body awareness in its fullness, you will know when you are in need in fundamental ways. Then you can choose your response.

—Hot and cold. These are often skin sensations, but there is a hot and cold that seems muscular and another hot and cold that seems "nervy," as one of my students termed it. Injured muscle that has spasmed and is releasing will sometimes become preternaturally hot, a heat that seems to subside as release is assimilated. This is a phenomenon which will one day be understood medically, I believe. In the meantime one comes to trust it experientially. It is always "good heat."

—Energy. Alexander Technique teachers vary across the widest possible spectrum with regard to "energy," from those who regard the use of the word in teaching as intellectually corrupt, indicative of a degenerate vitalism that has no place in the Technique, to those who champion "energy" as a breakthrough in teaching. There is a popular book on the Technique called *The Art of Changing*, by Glen Park. Its subtitle is *A New Approach to the Alexander Technique*. In it Glen Park advocates working directly with what she claims are energy systems in the body, particularly the chakra system, to add an energy support to the primary control.

Alexander Technique students likewise vary, from those who never use the word to describe their experience to those who use it constantly. When students never use the word it never becomes an issue. We simply proceed with their experience explored in kinesthetic terms. When students do use the word I try to find out what they mean. Very often they are using "energy" or "energy flow" as a kind of metaphor for kinesthetic qualities. If that is the case I help them name their experience more concretely. In the case of "flow," the student who first says, "I can really feel the energy flowing!" and then experiments with other language, "I feel flowing," "I am flowing," will generally find that the latter expression, "I am flowing," is more accurate and intimate. Flowing as a kinesthetic quality is under the student's control. If she wants to feel flowing she accesses her primary control. If she wants to diminish flowing she pulls down. If she's an actor she can even simulate pulling down while continuing to experience flowing.

Sometimes the students are experiencing energies that they have cultivated with practices like yoga. I tell those students that I am not adept at any of the practices that claim to cultivate energies and I probably won't be able to tell if the Alexander Technique is helping them with their practice beyond improving their use of their bodies. I invite them to determine for themselves what the relationship is between the energy that they enjoy and the primary control. Usually students report that their energy work is enhanced by the

Technique, and sometimes they report that their learning of the Technique is supported by their energy work.

Once in a long while a student is so habituated to thinking in terms of energy that she is unwilling to process kinesthetic experience. In every instance of this fixation that I have met there is a contempt for the body and bodily experience. Anything but "energy" is gross or disgusting or belies our putative status as spirits. Both the teacher and the student are challenged in this case. I suggest to the student that she go on experiencing whatever it is that she values *and* take a little nibble of embodiment just to see if she *might* like it.

There are three possibilities as I see it. One is that these "energies" that are mysterious and seem to be nonmaterial will one day be scientifically described, as was the stuff that knocked Benjamin Franklin to the ground when he flew his kite in a rainstorm. One is that they will come to be known as illusions. One is that they will be known to be imaginary but highly beneficial. As for Energy and the Technique, the debate continues.

Unified Field of Attention

I don't know if Frank Jones invented the phrase *unified field of attention* or if he borrowed it. In either case, he provided the Alexander community with a concept of critical importance. A unified field of attention is the ideal gestalt for Alexander learning, and it can be recovered. I say recovered because I believe we all had it as children. We lived as children within an attention in which we processed information from outside and information from inside at once. We did not split attention. We were not, as many people now are, either overly introspective or overly exterospective, neither of which states works well for Alexander learning. Both will destroy the integrity of artistic performance. An overly exterospective state excludes from awareness crucial kinesthetic information, and an overly introspective state fails to keep body feeling in contact with the world. Both states are uncomfortable to us. Both can be remedied. Simply do this. Whenever you notice that you have cut out half your experience by losing awareness either of yourself or of your world, simply open attention to the other half. Notice that your awareness of the one does not reduce because you have embraced the other. On the contrary, again and again students report that they see and hear more clearly when they are awake in their bodies or that their kinesthetic perceptions are enhanced when they open to space and time.

VII. Your Body Map and How to Correct It

The most valuable asset you can bring to the study of the Alexander Technique is an accurate body map. If your body map is inaccurate you can correct it. Body mapping work is work than you can do on your own once you understand what you're doing, and I promise you it will repay every minute you put into it.

William Conable developed the mapping work in his teaching of stringed instruments and the Alexander Technique at the Ohio State University. (For his account of his development of Body Mapping, see Appendix I, "Origins and Theory of Mapping.") He began to use mapping in his Alexander Technique classes and he discovered that it speeded learning of the Technique to a degree that he couldn't have predicted. My experience corroborates his. Mapping work is never instead of Alexander work. It is simply done at the same time, right in the course of hands-on work or work in activity.

It is because of the power of the mapping work that I use visual aids as much as I do in my teaching. Skeletons and anatomy texts are invaluable visual supports for a person's experience. A person will deliver weight efficiently into a chair through the rocker-shaped base of the pelvis if she can see a skeleton on the chair near her doing the same thing. Besides, it's fun.

The body map idea is simple and profound. Assume that you have a map of your body somewhere in your mind or nervous system or psyche or whatever you like to call the internal processing part of yourself that makes information available to you about you. Assume it is easy to gain access to your map. I have never asked a person a question about his body and not got an answer. If I say, "Where is the joint of your thigh with your pelvis?" or "What's a spine like, do you think?" or "Where are the joints with which you bow your violin?" or "Where are your lungs, anyway?" I always get an answer. Sometimes the answer is accurate and sometimes it is cloud-cuckooland and sometimes it's a little off. In any case the person will *always* try to move according to how he thinks he's structured. When there is a conflict between the map and the reality, the map will always win in movement. Perhaps that is Law of Human Movement III. When there is a conflict between the map and the reality, the map will always win in movement. Always. I have never seen an exception to it. It's inevitable because the map is what shapes our experience and we can change it only by a conscious effort.

Some mapping errors have career-destroying consequences. I have taught violinists and pianists suffering from tendinitis of the elbow. In my experience the malady is always caused by a misunderstanding of the rotation of the lower arm. If I say to the violinist, "Tell me about the rotation of the lower arm," I will always get an answer indicating that the rotation is around an axis on the thumb-side of the arm. And darned if they can't almost make it look like it works that way. The problem for them is that what they do to make it look that way tightens the muscles of the lower arm and puts a strain on the elbow joint that causes technical problems and injury. In fact, the rotation is around the bone on the little-finger side of the arm. When the violinist comes to understand the structure she will use the arm as it was designed to be used. Technical problems clear up and the tendinitis disappears because the pressure is off the joint. I discuss this in detail later in this chapter beginning on page 56. I offer it here simply as an illustration of the power of the map. William Conable has identified dozens of mapping errors, many of which have serious consequences in movement, this being only one.

The reason the mapping work is so effective in speeding Alexander learning is that students bring their faulty maps to the lesson and earnestly attempt to learn the Technique using the old map. Lessons alone may in time correct the map as the student achieves finer sensory appreciation, but the map still remains largely unconscious, whereas when the map is brought into consciousness and consciously corrected and refined the student has a cognitive tool that will go on improving her use of her body long after the lessons cease.

What follows in this section of the manual are pages that allow you to explore your map in ways that will assure that you bring an accurate map to your Alexander study. I have chosen these pages based on my experience of students and the mapping problems that most often contribute to confusion or misunderstanding as they learn the Technique. When the map is corrected the confusion clears and learning proceeds. The goal here is prevention and confusion-control.

If you want more detail, consider buying an anatomy book. Two that I recommend are *The Body Moveable* by David Gorman and *The Anatomy Coloring Book* by Kapit and Elson. See the bibliography for details.

I suggest that before you read further you take a few minutes and draw your body. A drawing of any size will do, and it can be a very simple drawing. Even if it is a stick figure or swirly and impressionistic you will be able to see in it salient features of your map. Keep your drawing handy as you read and check your drawing against the reality of these structures as you read so that you can be clear about where your map differs from your actual structure.

If you choose not to draw, then see if you can gain

access to the same information verbally. Ask yourself how you think about the structure in question. Say to yourself, for instance, "How do I think about my body? What do I think a human body is like?" You can simply imagine what you would draw, if you like, and then compare the image to the illustrations in the manual.

As you read, begin to explore the consequences of your map in movement. As you look down at this book, for instance, where do you imagine the joint to be at which you tilt your head? Are you simply tipping your head at the top of your spine, or do you bring your whole neck forward, too?

We must begin here with the statement of a fact that will seem absurdly obvious to some of you. If so, just bear with me and proceed, because what I am about to say will be crucial for a few of you, and I will risk offending the many for the few. There are three basic layers, onion-like, in our bodies: bone, then muscle, then skin. This needs to be said, because once in a while a person looks at her drawing and realizes that she sees no indication of a skeleton within. I have recently seen two such drawings. Both were made by women, which may be coincidence, and both women experienced a pervasive, burdensome over-work in muscles. One of the women, let's call her Julie, caught on immediately. As soon as she finished her drawing she exclaimed, "There are no bones in my drawing!" She continued to talk animatedly, "I think I'm a sort of mass, like a jellyfish. I really do think I'm like a jellyfish." Julie explored this aspect of her map for a whole morning. She drew another picture, resolutely including bones. She kept glancing at the full-size skeleton that was a feature of the room we were in. She shook her head from side to side and giggled as she drew. When she finished she held the new drawing in front of her and walked around the room feeling the reality of her weight delivering through her bony structure into the floor. Doing this she was able to simply let go of much of the over-work in her muscles. She said finding her bones, as she put it, was a great relief. The rest of us tried to imagine how we would feel if we had her map, 150 pounds of jelly holding itself up by sheer effort in the jelly, moving by bending the jelly. We decided we were very glad we weren't actually like that. By the end of the day Julie had a far more buoyant and articulated body. She had discovered bones were "neat."

Amy, the other woman with no bones in her map, did not have fun initially. Skeletons made her think of death. "I guess if I think I don't have bones in my body I think I won't have to die like all those people who foolishly have them." "Any truth in that?" I asked. "No." "Death is a big deal for me," she added. "Death is a big deal for everyone," I said. Amy didn't end the day thinking bones were neat, but she did end the day freer in her muscles and somewhat more comfortable in her mortal body.

One young man said it helped him to think of muscle as having function, as being there in order to move and stabilize bone. Muscle had existed in his map entirely for what he called its nuisance factor, its tendency to tense and cause trouble. His case illustrates in a strange fashion a feature of the map. The map contains structure and function. I quoted Patrick Macdonald's famous phrase, "The facts are friendly." Muscles have a function.

Others in that group came to appreciate the dual function of skin, as container and agent of contact, a kind of interface between our bodies and the world. Some had a sense of one function at the expense of the other. Those who had over-emphasized the contact function found they felt more secure when they also experienced their skin as boundary. Those who were "put in a basket bound with skin," to quote a song, enjoyed the skin's contacting function. They felt less isolated.

So, as you correct and refine your body map, give as much attention to function as to structure. Ask both, "What is it like?" and "What does it do?"

Alexander's "orders" to himself as he struggled to improve his use of his whole body were, "I wish my neck to be free so that my head may move forward and up so that my back may lengthen and widen." You will understand easily why Alexander chose those words if you understand that they describe a movement out of downward pull. If we wanted to teach a beautifully balanced person downward pull, we might give him "orders" as follows: "I wish my neck to tighten so that my head may pull down and back so that my back may shorten and narrow." The person would have to make this movement again and again until it became a habit he could chronically maintain. It would be hard to teach downward pull and hard to learn it. The student would have to think about it constantly and be really vigilant against his customary ease and freedom. To re-learn primary control is easy by comparison, first because it is re-learning and second because we cooperate with an inherent pattern rather than impose an arbitrary one.

To put an accurate map in place for learning Alexander's Technique let us turn first to the elements in Alexander's orders to himself. "I wish my neck to be free so that my head may move forward and up so that my back may lengthen and widen." You have already seen a picture in this manual of the muscles of the neck. Here is another view, exposing deeper layers:

Notice that the neck has a clear upper limit at the back—the base of the skull—and a clear lower limit in front—the collar bones. Those muscles surround the top seven vertebrae of the spine, so they are long. They are also big and powerful. They have to move a head, and a head is heavy. They are complex because head movement is complex.

The muscles of the neck are layered like artichoke leaves. Here is another layer:

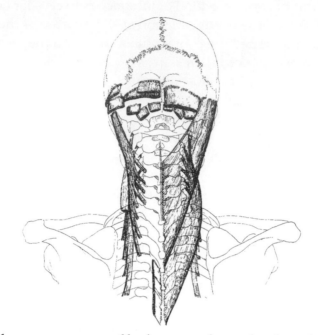

And interior to those are a group of little postural muscles that play an important role in the easy movement of the head forward and up out of downward pull, the ones you see below.

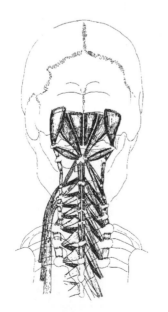

Now is the time to ask yourself the all- important question for correcting your map, "Is that how I think it is?" Say the word neck to yourself. What does the name conjure? Look at your drawing of your body. Does your neck look like what you see above? Is it a long structure? Is it powerful? Does it come all the way down to the collarbone? Is the neck in your map just in back? or does it come all the way around to the front, including all the way to the jaw? People who try to free their necks just in back get a very strange and unpleasant effect indeed, so this is important. A neck is all the head-moving muscles, front, back, and sides.

One of your best resources in correcting and refining your map is your finger-tips. Poke. Probe. Palpate. Right now run your fingers all along the base of your skull and feel where those muscles of the neck attach to the base of the skull. Some of you will instinctively reach several inches too low on the neck, which will tell you a great deal about how you think about your neck. If so, go on and on up with your fingertips until you find the actual bottom on your skull. There it is. As you run your fingers along the ridge where muscle meets bone you may feel that the muscles are tight there under the skull. If so, give them a loving rub. Notice that when you come all the way around to the ends of the base of the skull you are just behind your ear. Put a finger on the base of the skull and a finger in your ear so that you can feel that relationship. Then come on forward of the ear and feel the top of the jaw and gradually work your way down the jaw until you feel it angle forward, then follow it forward all along the horseshoe shape until your fingers meet. You have just palpated the upper limit of your neck, back (to the base of the skull,) sides (to the skull behind the ear,) and front (to the very bottom of the jaw.) Now run your hands all the way down your neck and run your fingertips back and forth along your collarbones. They are the lower limit of your neck in front. Now run your hands all over your neck again, front, sides, and back. Remember that interior to those muscles are the seven beautiful vertebrae of the upper spine.

Also interior to those impressive muscles of the neck is the throat. Necks move and support heads. Throats are the smaller structures within that speak and sing and swallow. When neck muscles tighten they not only pull the head off its poise on the spine, but they also exert a terrible tyranny on the small structures within; that tyranny was the source of Alexander's trouble with his voice.

If you find that your map of your own neck is inaccurate, just go into the part of your psychophysical being which contains your map and correct it. Some people do this readily and others need to learn to do it. Use any resource that works for you, drawing, feeling the part in question again and again with your hands, playing with movement in the part, looking in the mirror. When you take a shower run lots of hot water over your whole neck and soap it up luxuriously like a soap ad on TV and use the pleasure to help you with your map. Ask a friend to rub your neck. Xerox the pictures in this book eight or ten times and put them everywhere, refrigerator door, bathroom mirror, violin case, etc. When you come across one, say, "Ah, there's a neck."

One of the most useful things you can do is notice how the old map makes you move. Remember Law of Human Movement III: When there's a conflict between the map and the reality, the map always wins in movement. If you thought your neck was a sort of donut there between your head and your body, or like an O-ring, as some people tell me (some people even believe that the muscles go round and round their necks instead of up and down), then go back to that old, inaccurate map and notice how it makes you move. Tilt your head backward as if to look at the ceiling and notice how you compress your whole neck to preserve the donut image. Now correct your map. Remember the length of the muscles and where the top of the neck is. Make the movement again. Is it different? In what way?

Some people love to try to figure out how they arrived at their inaccurate map. Men often tell me that they read their necks off the mirror. The jaw hides the upper half of the neck, so only the lower half got credited. Worse, a shirt and tie hide the bottom inch or two of the neck muscles, and men learn to move as if the top of the collar were the bottom of the neck. These men will draw themselves with very short necks. A woman in her thirties brought me her beloved Barbie doll from childhood. Sure enough, the doll's head swivels from a joint just above collarbone level. The woman showed me how she rotates her head (no, rotated her head) exactly like her Barbie doll. Football players have demonstrated to me how they shortened their necks for protection when they played and then never quit shortening them.

Let's return to Alexander's orders and see where we are. "I wish my neck to be free so that my head may move forward and up so that my back may lengthen and widen." It is easier to free a neck, it seems to me, once one knows what a neck is. In downward pull the whole muscle group is habitually contracted. The degree of that contraction dictates the degree of consequent contraction in the whole body. So it is the whole muscle group that must be freed. How is it to be done? By intention. I have never met anyone with no ability to voluntarily free muscles. With practice that ability increases. But Alexander has made it easier for all of us by naming what occurs when we free—the head moves! What telling symmetry! When neck muscles tighten, the head moves. When neck muscles free, the head moves. Ah-ha! When the neck muscles tighten, the head moves down and back. When neck muscles free, the head moves forward and up. Back to the balance and poise on the spine that heads deserve. We have a coin with two faces, and it makes no difference whether you think heads or tails; you can think, "I will free my neck and therefore my head will move forward and up," or you can think, "I will allow my head to ease delicately forward and up and thereby free my neck." Makes no difference. Except that you have immediate feedback about whether you were successful. If you freed your neck, your head will have moved forward and up. If you released your head forward and up so as to re-establish its balance, you will have freed your neck. How will you know? It will feel freer. The muscles will be softer and longer and your head will feel more poised and balanced, and your back will have a chance to lengthen and widen out of its contraction, which nothing else but the freeing of the neck allows. But I am getting ahead of myself.

First we need to discover what a head is. Here is a picture of a skull:

And this is a jaw, which is appended to it. We have five limbs: two arms, two legs, and a jaw.

This distinction between the head and the jaw is crucial. A great many people have jaws in their maps. Two of them! A lower jaw and an upper jaw! This fantasy produces debilitating tension as the owners of two jaws attempt to move the upper jaw in relation to the lower, to feel equal movement in both. These folks laugh and laugh when they realize what they have been trying to do. Or, if they are singers, they may cry and cry. When they really get it that the upper teeth are in the skull, extraneous effort falls away. I'm convinced that this upper jaw fantasy contributes significantly to downward pull. The only way to feel as if the upper jaw is working is to move the head at its joint with the spine. To open the mouth then, the head has to move down and back.

Now, just as you palpated your neck, palpate your head. Run your fingers again along the base of your skull, then over your ear and then on forward along the cheekbone and down onto your top lip and top teeth. Everything north of there is head. You can tap with your fingertips all over your head.

Now please look at a picture of the base of the skull.

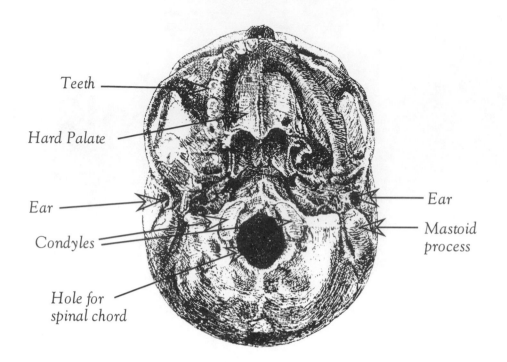

Teeth

Hard Palate

Ear

Condyles

Hole for
spinal chord

Ear

Mastoid
process

Notice it is a beautiful bony landscape with a hole in it for the spinal cord. This is where Yorick's head rests on Hamlet's hand. Notice that if you want to you can palpate nearly half of the base of your head with your tongue. Just run the tip of your tongue along your upper teeth and then back and forth over the hard palate. Then curl your tongue back onto the soft palate as far as you can go and the tip of your tongue will then be pointing toward the center of the base of your skull. Your tongue will be pointing right into the area of the joint of the skull with the spine, which is in the center of that lovely bony plain. It is there that a head moves forward and up—or down and back, for that matter. Rock your head, gently nodding, and feel the balance of the head on the spine—a sort of teeter-totter feel, front to back, back to front—as your head moves in relation to the occipital condyles.

An evolutionary perspective is invaluable here. We humans are the only vertebrates whose heads balance at the center between the front teeth and the posterior base of the skull, a feat which nature achieved slowly. The early hominids sported heads whose balance was forward of apes' heads and early Homo species balanced their heads progressively farther forward until in Homo Sapiens it is as you see, securing what paleoanthropologists call radical uprightness, our privileged position. If your body map tells you your head balances somewhere near the posterior base of your skull, your map is somewhere between one hundred thousand and several million years behind the times, depending on how far back the map says your head rests!

"I wish my neck to be free so that my head may move forward and up so that my back may lengthen and widen." Now we get to the crux. Here is a back.

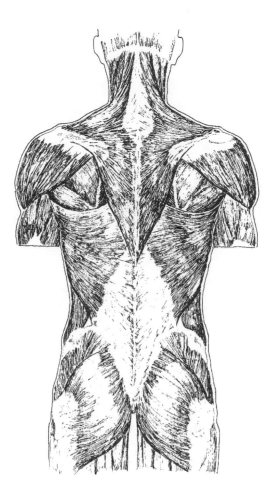

These muscles on the surface of the back are playing muscles primarily. Violin playing, racquet ball playing, basketball playing. They are muscles of expression. They can portray character or be wonderfully expressive in dance. They are designed to stay free and long so that they can make long graceful bow strokes and two and three point baskets and lovely gestures. But that is not their fate if neck muscles habituate tension. If neck muscles tense, so do these.

If neck muscles tense, the back shortens and narrows. Then in a bow stroke two kinds of work are going on, the work of shortening and narrowing and the work of bowing. Only the work of bowing is in the job description. Back muscles grumble, as well they should.

To clarify this matter further, look at the architecture of the bony structure again:

Notice again the centrality of our support. This is very important. There is a beautiful symmetry in the layering in the torso, front to back, or back to front: skin—movement muscles—support muscles—spine—support muscles—movement muscles—skin, with other body stuff like liver and heart and uterus tucked in amongst.

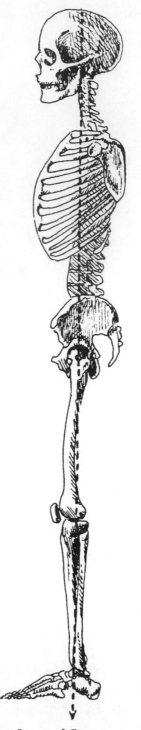

Line of Gravity

This is so important for learning Alexander's Technique because so many people have their torsos mapped inaccurately. Many people have their support mapped along the surface of their backs, like this:

These persons believe, "My back holds everything forward of it up." That's how they draw themselves, organized along their backs. What a terrible burden that puts on their backs, the parts of them designed to play violins and shoot baskets. When they comprehend the reality, "My spine and the support muscles that surround it hold up my back and my front," then they are able to allow their backs to lengthen and widen out of their habitual contraction so that the muscles that play violins and shoot baskets are free to do so.

What a bad design it would be if the support function were along one surface of us. I ask students what they would think if they looked outside and saw a tree significantly organized for its support along one side of the bark. What a bad idea! And yet some of them map their own trunks along one side of the bark and then wonder why standing and sitting are so tiring.

Look at your drawing and see if you have made your back do the work your spine is designed to do. Is your drawing organized around your back? Or have you drawn your spine on your back, as some people do?

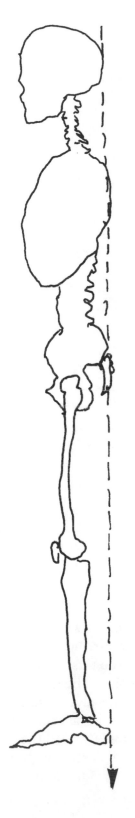

Here is a spine:

Front

Look at the design of the spine. I am going to repeat here what was said earlier because it is so important. The weight-bearing part of the spine is the front half. That is why only the front half has the little hydraulic pillows we call disks. Only the front half needs the cushioning of the little pillows.

Notice the long extensions on the back of the vertebrae. Those are called processes, and they are the source of much confusion. What I think happens is this. Johnny feels his own back with his fingertips and notices the bumps that are the ends of the processes under the skin. Or Johnny hugs Melvin and feels the tips of the processes under the skin on Melvin's back. The bumps get mapped as spine and, goodness gracious, are thought to bear weight. As Johnny unconsciously organizes his movement in keeping with his map, his back has to work hard to compensate for the loss of central support. The work gets interpreted as evidence that a back keeps Johnny upright! So a vicious cycle occurs in which the faulty mapping creates over-work and over-work confirms the map. The only antidote to this is the truth. Johnny's support is central. Johnny's back gets to ride the support of his spine and its postural muscles. Johnny can replace the faulty map with an accurate one and establish a virtuous cycle to replace the vicious one. As Johnny allows the work of up-rightness to leave his back, letting his back lengthen and widen, he feels the central support of his spine. The new freedom in his back confirms his accurate map. Virtue triumphs. "The facts are friendly."

Look at the skeletal structure again and notice that the *centrality* of weight-bearing pervades the whole architecture. It is at its center that the head delivers its weight on the spine. The spine's support is *central* to the torso. The arm structure suspends at the *center* of the ribs as seen from the side. The weight of the whole torso is delivered onto the leg at the *center* of the pelvis as seen from the side. Weight passes from the thigh bone to the lower leg at *center* and then the accumulated weight of the whole body is transferred through the foot into the ground at the *center* of the arch, delivering half the weight backward into the heel and half the weight forward into the rest of the foot.

My experience is that the arch of the foot must be accurately mapped before a student will really allow the freeing of the back in standing or walking. Classic downward pull almost always compels a person to put more weight on the heel in standing than on the front of the foot. Most people with that habit reflect it in their maps. They will tell you that weight is delivered at the ankle into the back of the heel and then forward into the rest of the foot. That's how it feels to them. Again, if this were true it would be a very bad idea. I think if it were true we would gratefully revert to being quadrupeds. Notice again how friendly the facts are. Our arches deliver weight from the center outward, like any arched structure, so the weight is transferred to the heel at its front and then backward through it into the ground. When the architecture of the ankle is respected and weight properly passes from the ankle backward into the heel there is a wonderful feeling of security in standing. There is a spreading of the bones of the foot forward of the ankle that is fan-like and gives a feeling of springiness, even in standing. When this occurs the toes are free for movement in a way they cannot be if weight is thrown onto the heel. (The toes are not part of the arch.)

Cutting the Pie in Squares

We suffer as a population from the devaluing of kinesthesia. One symptom, among many, of that devaluing is the ubiquitous faulty map, which we derive, at least in part, from this culture's odd naming of body parts. Consider, as an example, the word *waist*. The word *waist* stands as one of history's all-time Strange Categories. (If you are inclined to read a book about categories, read *Women, Fire, and Dangerous Things* by George Lakoff.)

The word *waist* dominates our mapping and therefore our moving. I say the word, and not the thing, because a waist is a fiction, a kinesthetic fantasy. Something arbitrary, and nothing anatomical, is named in the word waist. There is no cadaver in any medical school with a tag attached to a body part that reads "waist." Yet look at a roomful of people sitting and you will see that waist is the organizing feature of their sitting. Fewer than one person in twenty escapes by some mercy the treachery of a horizontal division of the body somewhere between the lowest ribs and the upper pelvis. The effect on movement of that division is incalculable. It makes people uncomfortable on car trips. It destroys support for singing. It cripples theatrical performances. It makes promising young athletes miss baskets. It makes attractive people dumpy. It belies the truth. The central organizing feature in the body is not horizontal, but vertical. It is the spine. The spine is not a fiction. The spine is real, and it does all the glorious things I have said it does and more. Persons organized around a spine move well. Persons organized around a waist are stuck.

To add insult to injury, we call our waist our middle. It is not. Our middle is the pelvic floor. We are divided in half at the hip joint. To regard the waist as our middle is to turn the pelvis into the upper part of the lower body, a kind of unit with the legs. This is the source of the stiff walking we see everywhere and of the odd maneuvers people make to pick up something from the floor. Do you remember how a toddler picks up something from the floor before she knows she has a waist? She bends at the ankle, knee, and hip joint. Her spine stays long and free. How, by contrast, do most adults pick up something from the floor? They stiffen their legs and try to bend at that fiction the *waist*, a movement which is ugly and dangerous. Young parents confide to me that they are so miserable after picking up toys in a room where a child has been playing that they often choose to live with clutter rather than do it. When they learn again how to bend where their child bends they enjoy the movement. And all because of a word.

We humans impose this torture only on ourselves. I once asked a veterinarian if she had ever heard anyone refer to a cat's waist, or a dog's, or a horse's. She said no, and she laughed. She thought it was a funny question.

The pelvis in fact the lower part of the upper body. The few persons who manage to defy their culture and retain the continuity of the torso—by torso I mean the long unit from the base of the skull to the pelvic floor—and who retain a pelvis oriented toward the spine in walking and standing and sitting, rather than toward the legs, have an enormous advantage over those who have succumbed to the waist-mystique. They tend to go to the top of their professions if they are athletes. Watch a tennis pro wait for a serve and you will see what I mean. Persons split at the waist have long since been weeded out by competition, and the pros bend at their middles, that is, at their pelvic floors, at their hip joints, and their spines retain their unity. The pros have the use then of all three leg joints—hip, knee, and ankle—and they can get around the court efficiently.

Look now at the drawing you made of your body. Is your waist the middle of the drawing? Is it the organizing feature of the body? Is the continuity of the spine obscured by that division? Does the pelvis orient toward the legs? If so, go look in a mirror and look at that organization in your body. What happens if you change your map? Find your middle at your hip joints. Shift to a spinal organization. Treat the spine as long and undivided. Allow your pelvis to find its relationship to the spine, to be a part of the torso.

Positions of Mechanical Advantage

I hope it is clear by this time that in Alexander work we are concerned equally with bone and muscle. We are searching out the most felicitous relationship among the bones in any activity, what Alexander called a position of mechanical advantage, and we want optimal support for those bones, the support which comes from muscles working in coordination, reflexly. Bones and muscle help each other. When we move our bones gently to a felicitous relationship we promote reflex support, and when we initiate reflex support by moving our heads forward and up and allowing our bodies to follow gently we encourage bones into a right relationship.

It is in achieving mechanical advantage that mapping helps us most. I am right now sitting in front of a computer as I write. I can be comfortable here for many hours if I bring my bones to a mechanically advantageous relationship with each other and if I do not interfere with their support. If I am uncomfortable I must figure out why I am uncomfortable and correct to comfort. I ask myself some simple questions: Is my head poised on my spine, or is it pulled forward of it? Am I allowing my front and my back to be equally supported on my weight-bearing spine? Am I allowing my pelvis to distribute weight into the chair efficiently? I may need to think about the structure of the pelvis and its relationship to the spine. I do not need fine detail, just accuracy and understanding of the simple mechanics of it. Here is a pelvis as seen from the side, showing its right relationship to the lumbar spine, those five large vertebrae just above the sacrum:

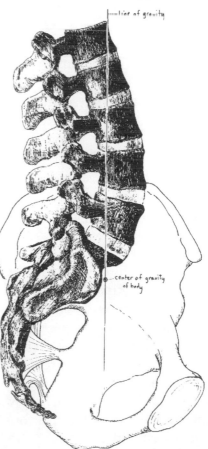

line of gravity

center of gravity of body

Notice that when we send our weight into a chair, we do so through bones shaped like rockers. Rockers are as good an idea for a pelvis as they are for a chair. The rockers of a rocking chair grant it mobility and uprightness at many angles. So it is with the rockers at the bottom of the pelvis. We may rock forward on them very far or back on them very far and they still send weight efficiently into the surface we are sitting on. Fine pianists, for instance, will often rock very far forward on those rockers when they play close to middle C, as do cellists when they go up the fingerboard (that is, closer to the floor!). These same cellists will often rock quite far back on the rockers as they come down the fingerboard. If the cellist's head is leading and her spine lengthening, that rocking backward can be a beautifully dramatic gesture to watch, and it gives a wonderful whole-body support to the left arm. Many people call those rockers their sit-bones, and many people have them oddly mapped. One cellist who used none of the mobility available to her at her rockers told me that her sit-bones were like spools. I could well imagine that I would not rock easily back and forth at the point of contact with my chair if I believed I had to balance on spools. When she correctly mapped the bottom of her pelvis she found she could feel beautifully balanced at any point on the rockers as she played, depending on what the musical passage required.

Notice also that the pelvis takes weight from the front of the spine through the sacrum at the sacrum's very top, where weight is directly sent into the pelvis from the sacrum. This leaves all but the top third of the sacrum free of weight-bearing, a lovely curving delta for protection and for pretty, as far as I can tell. Likewise the tailbone. Yet many people perceive themselves as sending weight into their chair through their sacrum and tailbone. They will tell you that they believe their weight goes through their tailbone and into the chair. Or through their tailbone into their sit-bones into the chair. The result is that they curl their pelvises down and back, putting an intolerable pressure on their lower backs. Notice that this is in keeping with the Third Law: where the map and the reality differ, the map wins. People throw weight onto their lower backs because that is what they truly believe they are designed to do. Thank goodness they aren't designed like that, really. Really weight goes through the pelvic structure into the chair, leaving the tailbone and most of the sacrum floating. Look at the structure from the front:

Think of what this structure means for standing. Again, "the facts are friendly." The top of the sacrum is thick to make it strong to take weight from the spine. Below that, the sacrum thins out. Similarly, the area of the pelvis that then sends weight into the hip joint is thick, like the thigh bone. If you have access to a skeleton, look at the pelvis and feel the thickness of that part of the pelvis. Notice that the pelvic bone thins above and below the weight-bearing area. The purpose of the thickened area is to send weight into the thigh bone, which has a curious and wonderful architecture to take weight quite far out to the edges of the body and then send weight down and in toward the knee. This gives humans a stability at the pelvic floor we could never have if the weight had to be borne farther in. Notice the line in the

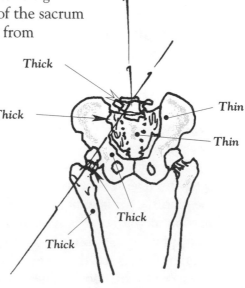

drawing that represents the delivery of weight in the pelvis, an angle familiar to us in buildings. An architect who took a workshop I did caught on right away. He said, "Why, the architect who first figured out how to handle the great weight of a cathedral dome must have been looking at a human pelvis!"

Notice that the pelvis is comprised of two bones that mirror each other. At the top, each meets the sacrum. At the bottom the two bones join at the pubis. Look at one of them from the outside:

Notice the location of the hip socket. Do you hear a recurring theme? The joint is at the center of the bone, in keeping with the centrality of weight-bearing laterally. It is here at the pelvic floor that our upper half meets our lower half. Our lower half —what we call our leg— has three joints—the hip joint, the knee, and the ankle—so as to distribute the weight of our upper half—our torso, head, and arm structure—efficiently, whatever position we are in. This may seem absurdly obvious to some readers, but others need to hear the obvious, for it differs from their maps. Many people consider the leg mobile at the hip joint who never think of the torso as mobile at the hip joint. If I ask those people to bend their torsos forward at the hip joint they can't do it, or they take a long time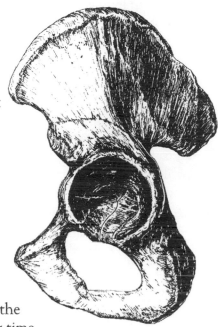
to do it, and it feels strange to them. Yet it is the most mechanically advantageous position for many of the things we do in life, like washing dishes. Look again (one cannot see too much of this) at F. M. Alexander in his mechanically advantageous position (*above, p. 10*), his upper half bent forward at the hip joint, and the joints of his legs positioned to easily handle the weight of his upper half. Alexander taught this relationship among bones directly—in Alexander jargon we call it "Monkey"—and it's a revelation to people who never bend forward at the hip joint, because when they learn monkey many activities become easy and natural for them that were stiff and difficult before, like waiting for a tennis serve or getting into their cars.

This mobility of the torso at the hip joints would be clearer to us, I believe, if we still squatted a lot. Suppose that like Bedouins we squatted to drink our coffee or suppose we squatted along rivers to wash our clothes or we squatted over little fires to cook our dals and chapatis. Squatting seems to be natural to humans, yet I find many of my students have lost the freedom to squat easily. Many can't squat with their feet flat. Even so, it feels good to them to do it, even for a very short time. Notice that squatting is simply a deeper Monkey. Think again about a little child picking up something from the floor. He squats, and the movement is smooth and always in proportion. The knees bend in proportion to the torso's coming forward. Good martial artists always exhibit that proportion. You can see it in kung-fu movies. The finest tennis players are in a half-squat as they wait for a serve. Imitate them when you see them. Play with squatting. If it's hard at first, it will get easier as you correct your map and regain primary control.

I often wish we didn't have the word leg in our vocabulary. If we only had the names of joints—knee, ankle, hip joint—we would move better. Many persons conceive legs as something to stand on more than something to move with. Most people will draw their arms with joints, or at least the suggestion of joints, but many draw their legs as sticks, with none of the leg's mobility indicated. When those persons come to sense their lower halves as articulated at joints in order to move, they move more freely. "Monkey" is a simple experiment in mechanical advantage. Learn it from your teacher and play with it a lot.

To add to the confusion, leg is for many persons that portion of the lower limb which lies between the knee and the ankle. My dictionary offers that as one definition of leg. The thigh portion of the lower limb is in this case relegated to a less prominent role in the map than it deserves.

Knees and ankles are often mapped so as to obscure their status as places where movement occurs. A person will often betray his map by his gestures. If he says, "My knees hurt when I stand for a while," he may accompany the words with a gesture, like cupping his knee caps in his palms, indicating that by knee he means knee cap. Then he may say, "Well, actually, it hurts behind my knee," confirming that knee for him is knee cap. When I invite him to reserve the word knee for the joint itself, there is a normalizing of the gait and greater ease in standing. The knee moves forward easily in walking, and the hamstrings lengthen rather than shortening. This is because every person who thinks of knee as knee cap tries to bend the knee at the center of the knee cap and focuses awareness on the front of the knee. The joint is actually at the bottom of the knee cap, as you can see by the picture, and should be felt in its whole circumference.

Kneecap

Knee joint

Likewise ankle. When I ask many people what they call ankle they put their thumb and fingers on the bumps that are the bottom of the lower leg bones. Those bumps are ankle in their map, and they earnestly try to move their feet from there. When they locate the joint itself, which is of course between the bumps, they immediately find it easier to move the foot and easier to balance over the arch. This clarity is crucial for learning the Technique. Remember that classic downward pull involves a shortening and tightening of the muscles of the legs in response to the shortening of the back and the pulling forward of the hip joint. This shortening alters the rest relationship of the lower leg to the foot, drawing the bones of the lower leg backward off the perpendicular at the ankle, at which point there is a muscular gripping at the ankle to compensate the loss of mechanical integrity. If a person releases out of downward pull in the neck and back and then does not allow a release out of the grip at the ankle there will be a dropping forward onto the front of the foot that is not comfortable. The release out of downward pull must bring the whole body out of its contraction, including the lower leg and foot, or there is a powerful incentive to go back to contraction. The releasing at the ankle will be difficult for the student who has the ankle mapped too high, or mapped as bumps, not joint. The map as you'll remember contains not just structure but also function. If a joint is mapped as joint, the implied function is movement. If the joint is mapped as bumps, movement in the area is not assumed. Some students look surprised if I ask them to move their foot at the ankle. If they are sitting they may reach down and feel the ankle and begin to tentatively circle the foot. "Oh, yeah, I guess it does move there. I never think of it that way." "How do you think of movement there?" "Well, I guess I think of movement in the foot—I can wiggle my toes— but I never think of movement *of* the foot."

Those students who do have the joint mapped as joint and therefore have no difficulty thinking of moving the foot at the ankle will sometimes nevertheless be unable to imagine moving the body at the ankle in relation to the foot, so the release back to the perpendicular of the leg bones at the ankle will feel strange to them. The movement will seem not possible, so they keep their ankles stiff. Do you see the similarity with the issue of the torso moving at the hip joint? Same problem, different location.

Mechanical advantage, then, is both the easiest distribution of weight at the joints and easiest mobility. The rest relationship of any joint is that relationship from which movement is easiest. The head moves easily when it moves from a poise on the spine. The torso and legs move easily from a poise on the arch. The torso moves easily from a poise on the legs. If the rest relationship is compromised by downward pull, to that degree movement loses its ease. We regain mobility by regaining the easy balance of bone in relation to bone. Here again in the wonderful reciprocity of muscle and bone is displayed a virtuous cycle. We free our muscles and the bones come home to rest; we bring our bones to right relationship and we free muscle for mobility and support.

The Happy Mapping of Arms

I have left discussion of arm mapping till last because I truly believe that they were an afterthought in the design, added on so that singers could have accompanists. They are slung over a balanced structure in a beautifully balanced way, and we are only in trouble with arms when we interfere with that balance. The prime agent of interference is—guess what?—classic down-ward pull. To be clear about how that interference occurs we once again turn to the structure. Here is an arm as seen from the front.

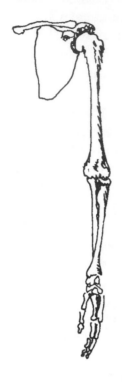

Notice that an arm includes a collarbone, a shoulder blade, an upper arm bone, two lower arm bones, a wrist, and a hand. The collarbone and shoulder blade are of importance here, because their inclusion in the arm means that there are four arm joints, not three as many people assume. The only place that the arm structure joins the torso *at a joint* is where the collar-bone meets the breastbone. At that joint the move-ments are available that we usually call raising the shoulders or bringing the shoulders forward or pulling the shoulders back or dropping them. If you place your fingers along your collarbone and make those move-ments you will see what I mean. The collarbone is moving in relation to the breastbone. The action at that joint can be clearly felt because the collarbone lies just under the skin. If you place your fingertips on the collarbone near the end where it joins the shoul-der blade and do the movements of raising your shoulders, bringing your shoulders forward, dropping your shoulders, pulling your shoulders back, you will find your fingertips moving with the collarbone in swoopy circles. If you then place your fingertips on your upper shoulder blade as you do those movements you will learn how much the shoulder blade moves, and how good it feels to let it move. The accurate mapping of the joint of the collarbone with the breastbone is critical for free upper torso and arm movement. If that joint is not mapped it is not used. It is held rigid and does not contribute its share of movement when it is needed, as in shooting baskets, or reaching for a cup on an upper shelf, or going to the upper string on the violin. This forces a disproportionate movement onto the second arm joint, the joint of the upper arm with the shoulder blade. That disproportion is a source of strain in activities that require repetitive use of all four arm joints, like swimming.

To make matters worse, much worse, actually, the people who believe they have only three arm joints usually misconceive the location of the first. If the arrows on the left reveal the truth, the arrows on the right reveal the fantasy.

Right:
4 joints

Wrong:
3 joints

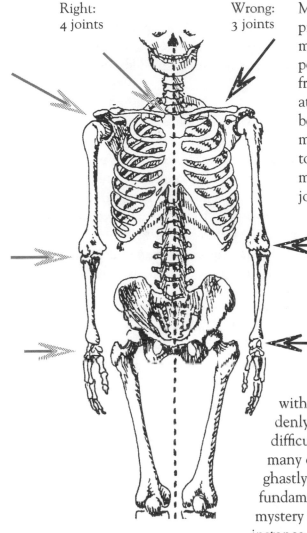

Many people share this mapping error and its attendant misery. Not only do these people not get the benefit of the free use of the actual first joint at the collarbone and breastbone, but they also tighten muscles in the whole upper torso to feel like they are moving at the imagined first joint, which as you can see is directly between the two real ones. Very nasty long-term arm problems can be cleared up by the simple expedient of the truth. I have seen looks of astonishment and delight on the faces of violinists who at last have the right number of joints to play with, in the right location. Suddenly bowing maneuvers that were difficult seem easy. In this case, as in many others, I often think what a ghastly waste it is that we keep the fundamentals of our structures a mystery to ourselves. Violinists, for instance, could be taught the simple arithmetic of their structures in their very first lessons, and then they wouldn't have to suffer because the calculus of their technique goes off when the arithmetic is wrong.

Why is the accurate mapping of the arms so important for learning the Alexander Technique? Because in the Technique we are interested in allowing the body to resume its native stature. If the body is shortened and narrowed by downward pull, we seek to allow it to lengthen and widen back out to its proper proportions. This will often involve a tremendous release out and up in the upper torso, because downward pull drew the upper torso down and in. No one will fully allow that releasing up and out who has mapped a joint somewhere between the real first and second arm joints, because the tension itself maintains the sensations of the illusory structure. There's a chicken-egg question here I don't know how to resolve. Did the tightening confirm the map or did the map derive from the tightening, or both? I don't know the answer, and I don't know how to find the answer, but it doesn't matter practically, because when a person exchanges the illusion for the reality, everything frees in keeping with that change. Then, when an Alexander teacher guides a movement for her student that facilitates that release up and out of the upper torso the student has no trouble following her because the movement does not defy, as it did before, everything the student believed about that part of her.

You may wonder why I say upper torso when I could say shoulder, which is one word instead of two. Because I believe the framers of the English language gave us in the word shoulder a word nearly as destructive of good moving as the word waist. Another instance of dividing the pie in squares, which can be done, but which betrays good sense. In a roomful of ten people, if I ask them, "What is a shoulder?" I will get at least four or five different answers, and two or three of them will be mutually exclusive, whereas in answer to the sensible question, "What is a nose?" there would be unanimity. The most common answer with regard to shoulder is one which includes about a third of the collarbone, about a quarter of the shoulder blade, a couple inches of upper arm, and a bite of two or three ribs. That makes no sense! I tell my students to delete the word shoulder from their body vocabulary (they may need the word on the highway) for at least the next six months and to think instead in terms of their arm joints. If one has shoulders, those things stuck up there on top of us somehow, it is impossible to figure out where they go. If one has arm joints, on the other hand, it is perfectly clear where they belong at rest.

Where? Where do they belong? The first joint—that joint of the collarbone and breastbone, remember—is at its rest relationship when the collarbone is roughly parallel to the ground. It is neither too far up nor too far down, neither too far forward nor too far back, but just balanced. In some people the collarbone has been pulled so far down and back that it has nearly disappeared, a serious problem for violinists because the collarbone is the violin shelf. A serious problem for dancers because it makes upper torso movement ugly. When the collarbone comes back to its rest position there will be a feeling of ease, and movement will be available in all directions from that joint. Do you see that again and again mobility is the key? If it's free, it can move.

The second arm joint, the joint of the upper arm with the shoulder blade, must be mapped correctly in order to completely free the back. Here we are up against not only the ubiquitous faulty map but a major bit of cultural conditioning—the posture thing. The P-word. A central tenet of the posture dogma is "Get your shoulders back," or the harsher version, "Get those shoulders back." I sometimes want to cry when I see a student who has obeyed that commandment for decades, always hurting between his shoulder blades, never feeling a free movement of arms. Surely daddy and mommy and grandma were right! No, daddy and mommy and grandma were wrong, wrong, wrong. Shoulders don't belong back. God didn't design them that way. The second arm joint is designed to balance at the very center laterally. Sound familiar? At the center. Neither forward, nor back, but just balanced at center. Take a look.

A View of the Ribs from above:

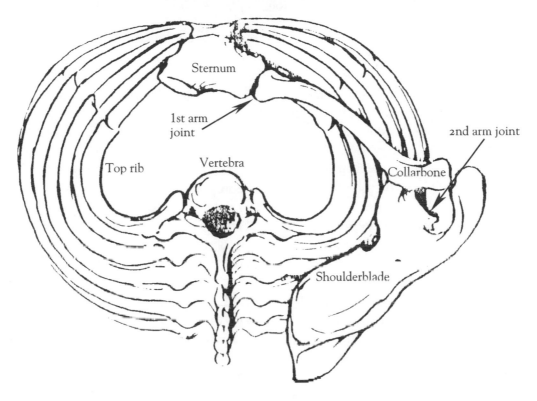

Daddy was wrong. Mommy was wrong. No shoulders back. Shoulders back makes children miserable and it makes adults miserable and it destroys the careers of musicians. It also makes learning the Alexander Technique more taxing than it need be. Students sometimes have a hard time getting it that we really don't teach posture, that Alexander bears no relationship to the posture thing. We teach a different Head Up, the one that frees, not the one that stiffens, not the Head Up followed by Shoulders Back. This is particularly important for the student to understand who in fact carries her arm structure forward of center, because she will feel as her head moves back to its poise on her spine and her spine lengthens out of its shortening that her arm structure is easing back home. She will love how this feels, the freedom of it, and she is in danger of trying to reproduce the feeling she liked by moving her arm structure without the prerequisite freeing upward of the spine, in which case she gets not freedom but strain. She is very likely to call the freeing an opening, and she may make a gesture indicating width across the front of her. This too is dangerous if she attempts later to achieve an opening in front at

the expense of a closing in back. She may be so used to narrowing in back
that she doesn't notice the tightening, though she will know she is missing
the good feeling she had under the teacher's guidance. If the student correctly
maps the second arm joint so that she is looking for that sense of balance and
ease rather than for placement or posture or openness, she will have a clarity
about the widening of the back, which allows the arm structure to ease back
to balance.

The Lower Joints of the Arm

If you are a musician with tendinitis of the wrist or elbow, or if you have
problems with finger control, or if you suffer from carpal tunnel syndrome or
tennis elbow, then you should pay careful attention to the structure of the
two lower joints of the arms and correct your map if necessary. I can almost
guarantee that your map will be incorrect if you
experience those difficulties.

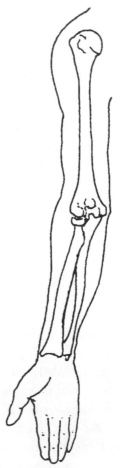

Let's examine the elbow joint first. It is a joint of two
bones with one, as you see in the picture. There are
two bones in the lower arm in order to make it
possible to rotate it to bring a violin into playing
position. (Perhaps it will be clear to you by now that
the structure of the whole body can be explained by
the necessity to arrive at a violinist, which I think of
as the Creation Imperative or the Evolution Imperative, take your choice.) Kidding aside, if all we did
with the lower arm were open and close it, we would
only need one bone in the lower arm. But we also
rotate the lower arm. Notice that it is a different
rotation than is available at the shoulder joint,
where there is also a rotation available (with a
different design not requiring two bones). Play
with both rotations until you have them completely separated in your experience.

Violinist, when you bring your violin up to
playing position you are making two movements at the elbow. You are bending at the
elbow and you are rotating at the elbow. It is
misunderstanding the rotation that gives so
much grief. Violinists in trouble almost
always shorten the lower arm in that rota-
tion because they believe that the rotation occurs around an axis on the
thumb side of the lower arm. Oddly enough, they can almost make it look as
if it does, but nonetheless it doesn't. The axis in the rotation is the bone on
the little finger side of the lower arm.

Study the illustration here
which shows exactly how that
rotation occurs. I will guide you
through a series of explorations
that will allow you, I hope, to
perceive this clearly in your own
body.

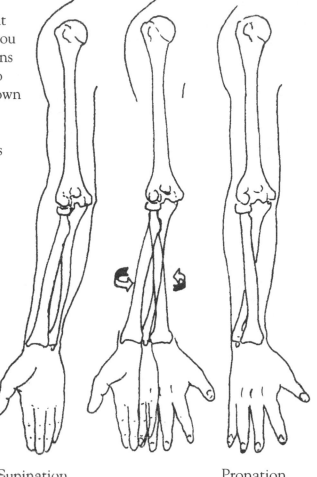

Begin by running your fingers
along the bone on the little
finger side of your lower arm.
That bone is called the *ulna*,
and it is easily felt in its
entire length. You will find
the lower end of it by
beginning with the quite
discernible bump just
above your wrist. That
bump is the base of an
arm bone. (Once in a
while I meet someone
who calls that bump and
the one on the other side
the wrist. If you do that,
please change your map.
Your wrist is between
those bumps and your

Supination   Pronation

hand.) The other end of the ulna is the point some people call the elbow.
Run you fingers up and down the ulna many times until its location is utterly
clear to you. Then switch your attention to the other lower arm bone, the
radius. Locate the lower end of the radius by finding the corresponding bump
above the wrist on the thumb side. Follow that bone up the length of your
lower arm. At the upper end it will be difficult to feel, because the muscle is
thick there, but you can do it. Hold your arm parallel to the floor with your
palm up. With the thumb and fingers of your other hand feel both bones at
once. You will find that in this position they are parallel to each other.

Now discover what happens in the rotation. Still with one palm facing the
ceiling, lay the fingers of your other hand along the length of the ulna.
Stretch the examining fingers a little if necessary so you can feel the whole
bone. Gently rotate your lower arm. Notice that the ulna doesn't turn. The
fingers of your examining hand stay in the same place while the palm of the
rotating hand turns to face the floor as a result of the rotation of the lower
arm.

Now you know something important. The ulna is the axis in the rotation, the stable thing around which everything else moves. About the word *axis*: because the earth turns on a axis at its center, some people conclude that where there is rotation the axis must be central. Not so. We might call the binding of a book its axis. That axis would then be central to the book, but it lies in relation to each page as the ulna does to the rotating arm, along one side. Notice that the rotation of the lower arm is not 360, but 180 degrees, like the pages of most books. That's because that's sufficient rotation to bring a violin up. The Creation Imperative did not require more rotation.

Now change the position of your examining hand. Place your middle finger on the upper end of the ulna and your thumb on the upper end of the radius. Again rotate your arm. Notice that your examining thumb and finger stay in the same place. Nothing is happening there either! What, then, can account for the movement? The mystery is about to be solved. This time place the tip of an examining finger on the *lower* end of the radius and rotate. Ah, do you see? Your finger travels the 180 degrees with the lower end of the radius, so the radius is simply crossing the ulna in the rotation. Do you see? The bones which are parallel before the rotation are crossed afterward: one has crossed the other. Now take two pencils or two table knives or your two index fingers and make them stand in for the bones of your lower arm so you can represent this phenomenon to yourself in another way. So, hold up your index fingers parallel to each other and nearly touching. Now simply lay the right finger, which is the stand-in for the radius, over the left finger, which is the stand-in for the ulna, to form an X. The ulna remains stationary and the radius moves in relation to it. That's how the bones of the lower arm work in rotation.

What's the big deal? The big deal is—and it is a very big deal: musical careers crash and burn because of it—some players have it backward. Some players try to stabilize the radius and move the ulna around it. They treat the thumb and the thumb side of the lower arm as an axis and they earnestly attempt to bring up a violin around it. Thereby they seriously tense the lower arm muscles and put an eventually intolerable strain on both the elbow and the wrist.

There are some other clues to this malady besides the tensing of the lower arm. One is the orientation of the hand. Those who map the rotation incorrectly almost always keep the thumb on a line with the radius at rest. That is how their hands rest in their laps. That is how they reach for a doorknob or a faucet. That is how they wave good-bye or extend their hands for a handshake. If I've described your habit, take some time to examine the habit. Bring your hand to that habitual relationship with the arm (the thumb lined up with the radius) and slip your thumb in under your palm. With the thumb hidden in this way it may be clearer that your habit angles your hand in relation to your arm in such a way that there is a chronic contraction across the outside of your wrist. Now, strange though it will feel, move your hand so that your little finger lines up with your ulna. Now hide your thumb under your palm and you will see that the hand is in a easy relationship with the arm that does not involve a chronic contraction on either side of the wrist. That is the rest relationship of the hand to the arm, the relationship from which movement is easiest. Most people keep their hand in that relationship to the arm unless there is a need for movement at the wrist. Rest position is a good clue to the map.

The Wrist and Hand

Here's an irony. A number of people who have come to me with serious use-induced problems in their wrists or hands don't even *have* a wrist in their body maps. They draw their hands meeting their arms at the location of the wrist. Several of those people, though, had their knees mapped as things, drawn as big round circles between the thigh bone and the lower leg, often with a bitty-little kneecap drawn in front of it. I surmise that the pressure on their knees from downward pull had made the knees feel as big as soccer balls but that the shortening of the arm structure had distorted kinesthetic perception differently in the wrist so that the wrist wasn't even perceived. This is another instance in which a person with a mismapping can make the body appear to be structured as they imagine it to be. These people looked as if they had no wrists.

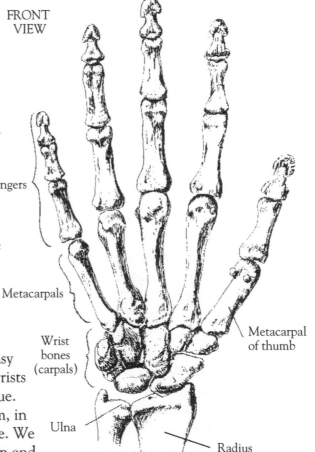

FRONT VIEW

Fingers

Metacarpals

Wrist bones (carpals)

Metacarpal of thumb

Ulna

Radius

Here is the wrist. It is very easy to say what we are after for wrists with the Alexander Technique. We want no pressure on them, in particular no chronic pressure. We want a long easy sweep of skin and muscle and tendon across the joint, and we want full mobility with no retracting across the joint in movement. We want the fingers to move without the wrist stiffening, even to grip or strike. For dancers and actors we want the wrist eloquent. In order to achieve the freeing of the wrist it needs to be accurately mapped.

Notice that the first joint of the thumb is at the wrist rather than at the end of a metacarpal. Chronic tightening of the wrist loses the thumb its mobility in relation to the other fingers and then the thumb will not lie easily in the palm as it should. So, free your wrist, free your thumb.

The Continents of the Body

Most people come to the Technique with a map the large-scale divisions of which (the continents, if you will) are: Head-Neck; Above Waist; Below Waist; Arm; Arm; Leg; Leg. The waist serves as a kind of Panama Canal in that geography, dividing the developed world from the undeveloped. Legs are purely Third World. I recommend a new world order: Head; Torso; Arm; Arm; Leg; Leg; Jaw.

I hope you can see that the mapping work is fun as well as effective. You can do it mostly on your own, using resources like the anatomy books I named at the beginning of the chapter, though your teacher will help you. Once you have your map accurate in the location of the joints and the mechanics of weight-bearing you can go for almost infinite refinement, if you like. You may want to have great detail in your map for particular purposes. I know an oboe player who has a detailed understanding of the muscles in her cheeks which enables her to make subtle changes in embouchure which allow for wonderful variety in the sound. Some singers have a complex map of the vocal mechanism and can change the shape of the area beneath and behind the soft palate at will in order to get just the vowel sound they want. Actors may not need great detail in the structure aspect of their maps, but they will need sophistication with regard to function. I told my theater movement class that they should be able to wiggle their scalps and their ears. Some of them thought that was silly till one handsome young man in the class demonstrated that his Joe College grin could be made to look completely gooney simply by pulling his ears back while he did it. That grin could land him a comic role that the non-ear-wiggling actor couldn't get. Daniel Day Lewis got an Academy Award for, among other things, the mobility of his left foot.

There is a body work called Body-Mind Centering developed by Bonnie Bainbridge Cohen which must be mentioned with regard to mapping and body awareness. Cohen invites her clients to feel in their bodies all sorts of things which I find it hard to believe that anyone can feel, like the spleen or the flow of lymph or the making of cells in the marrow. I can't myself feel any of that, and I don't know if I could learn to. Cohen's students claim they have learned to. If so, then a map can be even more refined and even more completely experienced than I know. Certainly, when I began to recover kinesthesia I didn't have a clue that a mere twenty-nine years later I would be able to feel all that I can now feel. Which is to say, in the matter of mapping and awareness, assume no limits, and play.

The Useful Mapping of Muscle

Most of the early work on body mapping focused on the skeleton because people suffer so much from misunderstanding and therefore mis-using their joints. It was clear to both Bill Conable and to me that there were mapping issues with regard to muscle, but we were not in the beginning able to discern more than three rudiments.

First, there were instances in which students simply needed to know that muscle existed or that it did not in certain locations. People who believe, as many earnestly do, that their fingers are covered with muscle are constantly producing effort in the fingers to justify the map. What relief when they find out it isn't true! Conversely, people who believe that skin rests on bone in their faces have mask-like faces and only regain real mobility and facial expressiveness when they discover the complex layer of muscle that lies between bone and skin in the face. Many beginning Alexander students believe they move their heads with muscles on their heads or in their heads and can learn to free their necks and allow their heads to be light and mobile only when freed from the horrible illusion of massive head muscles.

The second rudiment was the already mentioned all-important distinction between voluntary action and involuntary action in the muscles. When students tried to feel the involuntary work of staying upright in the same way they feel voluntary movement—as the sensation of movement—rather than as movement quality—balance, buoyancy, poise—they were in trouble. Voluntary action in muscle can be done; involuntary action in muscle must be allowed, permitted, cooperated with, encouraged, coaxed. This distinction lies at the heart of the doing/non-doing paradox in movement.

The third rudiment was that usefulness in muscle mapping probably depended on an understanding of muscle groups. In downward pull we tighten the head-moving group of muscles and we must free the group in order to get out of downward pull.

Beyond that it wasn't clear what was useful in muscle mapping. Students who took anatomy and cut up cadavers and gained high marks in their physiology classes were not necessarily better off in their bodies. They were lost in the complexity or the particularity of it, unable to see the forest for the trees. They were troubled by a tight this or a tight that without any hope of freeing the tight this or the tight that. The tight muscle was mapped but the map wasn't usable, like having a map of treasure island but no boat.

Now someone has come along with a boat. Joan and Alexander Murray in Champaign-Urbana, Illinois, became interested in the work of the late anthropologist Raymond Dart, who studied human evolution with emphasis on primate structure and its progress toward uprightness. Dart developed a set of positions of mechanical advantage based on what he had learned, and the Murrays have used Dart's procedures, as they are called, to further Alexander learning in much the same way that Alexander teachers have always used the "monkey" position.

In Dart's writing* there is much truly useful discussion of the spiral organization of the musculature. Dart's descriptions of the muscle structure expand and refine the rudiments mentioned above at just the right level of abstraction. He says: this muscle group lies here on the skeleton and it works this way and this is why. His descriptions are neither too simple nor too detailed to be useful. They meet the criterion of good mapping in that the information alone improves body use as soon as it is comprehended. Further, Dart's procedures used in the context of Alexander's discoveries build a bridge between the voluntary and the involuntary that provides the firmest possible foundation for complex movement.

When bone is mapped as bone it is the space between bones that becomes most important. We love joints. Next best is weight bearing, the wonderful feeling of support that comes from easy delivery of weight through the bones. The useful units of the bony structure are suggested by those two factors, joints and weight delivery.

A shift of attention to muscle groups suggests another topography. We are used to this with regard to other maps, and we need to get comfortable with it with regard to the body map. Example: we know that if we look at a map of North America that shows bodies of water it will look different from a map showing elevation or wind currents, yet each is accurate. Similarly, the bone map and the muscle map will organize the same space differently. Take the pelvis, for instance. I have made a strong case for thinking of the pelvis as part of the torso, the lower part of the upper half of the body, the pelvic floor being our middle.

The same territory seen from the point of view of the muscle groups suggests a strong emphasis on the spiraling of muscle from the buttocks down around the thigh to the knee, supporting a view of the pelvis as part of the legs. No reason to choose one over the other. Each view is accurate and each view has its usefulness. What I have here called buttock muscles are regarded as lower back muscles by the map suggested earlier in the book. It is very useful to regard those muscles as lower back muscles because it makes it utterly clear that they are as subject to narrowing when the neck muscles tighten as are the muscles of the upper back. To shift perspective and see those muscles as buttock muscles in relation to the muscles of the thigh is to see the reality with an eye to the inevitable tightening of the thigh and loss of mobility at the hip joint when buttock muscles tighten. Both are useful perspectives. No

---

* Consult John Coffin's bibliography at the back of the book for references to the Dart work. I especially recommend Skill and Poise.

need to choose. Is the Ohio River the top of Kentucky or the bottom of Ohio? Yes. You can have your cake and eat it, too. If you regard the pelvis as the lower part of the upper body you will be much more likely to balance the upper half of you beautifully at the hip joint. If you regard the muscles that cover the rear of the pelvis as in some important way continuous with the thigh muscles you will allow a release of the whole spiral to the knee. Two for the price of one.

VIII. Breathing Free

In the early years when F. M. Alexander taught in London he was known as "the breathing man." We could still call his technique "the breathing technique," so great is its contribution to breathing. "I can *breathe*," is a frequent report from students about their experience as they learn the Technique. A recent study confirmed what we teachers see every day. Dr. John H. M. Austin, a chest radiologist from Columbia-Presbyterian Medical Center, gave tests to subjects before and after a series of Alexander Technique lessons. The results showed "significant increases" in the tested qualities, particularly rib mobility and vital capacity. The article was published in the journal *Chest*, under the title "Enhanced Respiratory Muscular Function in Normal Adults after Lessons in Proprioceptive Musculoskeletal Education without Exercises." Austin describes the Technique as a way of gaining "awareness and voluntary inhibition of personal habitual patterns of rigid musculoskeletal constriction."

The improvement in breathing that always results from successful Alexander lessons has two sources. The first is eliminating the interference of the downward pull on breathing and the second is accessing optimal reflex support for breathing.

In this chapter I invite you to help yourself and your teachers by correcting your body map of the territories of breathing. This assumes your map is incorrect. Forgive me if you are an exception. If so, you should consider yourself a most fortunate human being, for most people have egregiously inaccurate maps of the breathing territories and they suffer as a result.

We'll begin with the lungs, because the rest of the mechanism of breathing makes sense in its relationship to them and because so many people have their lungs so strangely located in their body maps, like Pike's Peak in Vermont. The lungs actually live in the thoracic cavity, which as you can see by the picture is about the upper half of the rib area and about the upper third of the torso. The heart is nestled in between the lungs, and just below the lungs and the heart is the diaphragm, which is shown on this picture as the wavy line separating the thoracic and abdominal cavities.

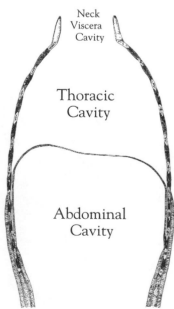

Neck
Viscera
Cavity

Thoracic
Cavity

Abdominal
Cavity

Here is a picture of the lungs *in situ*, as seen from the front. You will see the lungs from the back and from the sides on subsequent pages. Some things to notice: the top of the lung is above the collarbone, the bottom at about the bottom of the sternum; the nipple is at about the widest part of the lung; the lungs fill the part of the rib area that is continuous, all around; the part of the rib area that houses digestive organs is not continuous all around, but sports the inverted V that is the very handsome upper abdominal wall; the diaphragm is NOT the same as the upper abdominal wall.

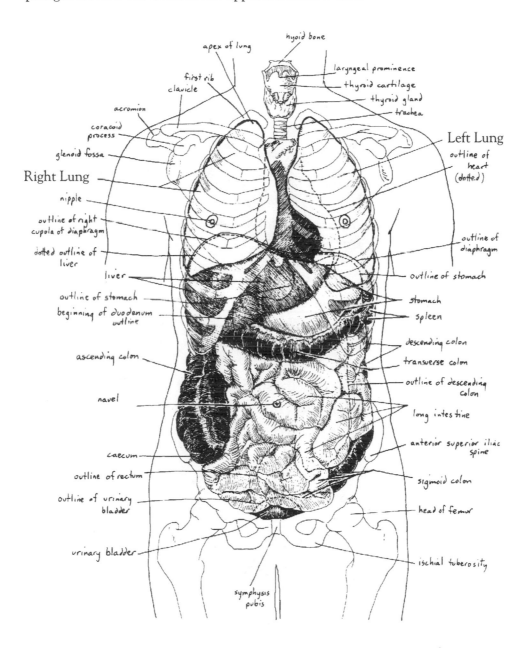

Here are the lungs as seen from the back. Some things to notice: a shoulder blade acts as a shield, significant protection for each puncturable lung, along with the ribs. Each rib makes a joint with a process on a vertebra, so you can see your twenty-four breathing joints in this picture. (The narrowing of the back constricts those joints.) The floating ribs, which lie below the level of the lungs, are compressed and pulled forward when the back shortens and narrows in downward pull; as the back lengthens and widens the floating ribs get to float back where they belong.

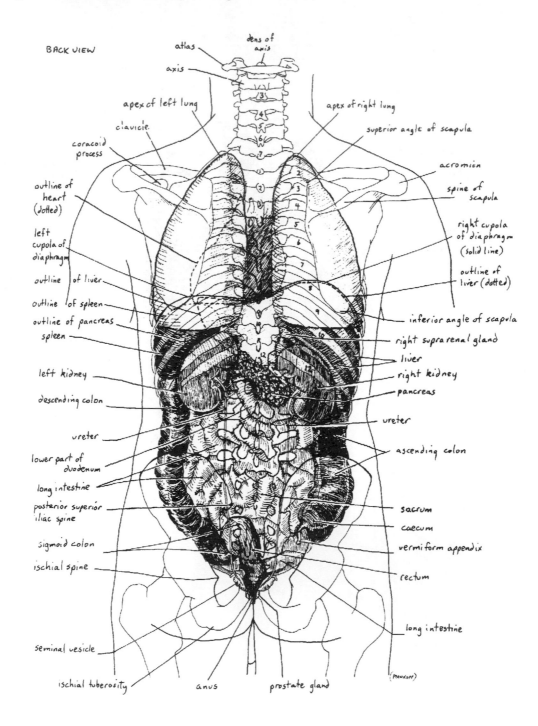

Here the lungs are seen from the side. Some things to notice: the bottom of the lung is at the same level as the bottom of the breast. All breast tissue overlies ribs. The ribs angle down from back to front and each rib is continuous from its joint with the spine in back all the way around to the cartilage in front, so in rib movement each rib acts like a bucket handle as it comes up and out on inhalation and down and in on exhalation. Notice that ribs are as individual as fingers. Notice that there is muscle between ribs (what you eat if you eat spareribs). Those muscles, called intercostals, are responsible for about a quarter of the muscular work of breathing.

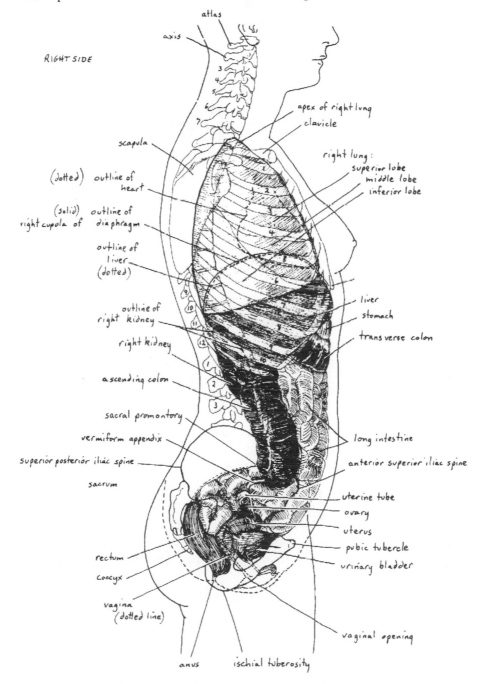

Now let's put the lungs in the context of the rest of the torso. This middle section of the torso is called the abdominal cavity. The abdominal cavity houses your liver, stomach, and spleen, that is, digestive and other stuff. The diaphragm is a dome, and there's a picnic going on under it. The southerly portion is called the pelvic cavity, and it houses eliminative and reproductive functions. No air goes into the abdominal or pelvic cavity in breathing. There is plenty of movement in these areas in breathing but no air, so if someone invites you to feel air in the lower two-thirds of your torso try to find out what it is the person is looking for. People who talk that way are using the word *air* not literally but metaphorically. Probably they are looking for more movement. Try to find out.

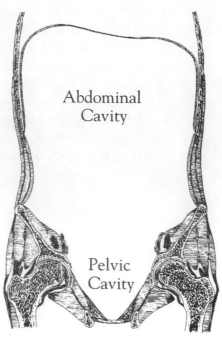

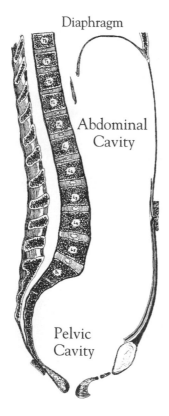

Here's another perspective on the same territory, a side view. Please notice again the vast range of the torso into which no air may go. This territory is for other things, including the structures that support breathing. One of my students noted recently how wonderfully reassuring it is that support for breathing is *underneath* the diaphragm and the air rather than in front of it or alongside it. Notice the great length of spine available for lengthening on exhalation and the great depth of the pelvic cavity. This view provides another opportunity to admire the spine. The bottom five vertebrae comprise the lumbar area, which curves forward. They are part of your support of singing, speaking, and breathing.

Next let's go to the second most mismapped breathing structure after the lungs, the diaphragm. You have already seen the diaphragm's location indicated by a line. Here is the whole muscle from two perspectives. On the left the diaphragm is drawn from above and behind; on the right it is drawn from

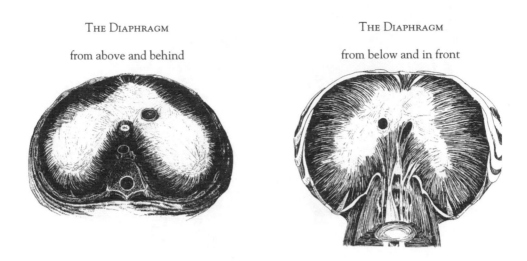

THE DIAPHRAGM

from above and behind

THE DIAPHRAGM

from below and in front

below and in front. Notice that the diaphragm is a horizontal structure. It is most commonly mismapped as vertical, like the abdominal wall. Indeed, quite a few people have the diaphragm and the abdominal wall confused, and they will put their hands on the abdominal wall in an attempt to palpate the diaphragm. Some of my students have told me that it is called the diaphragm because it is the same size and shape as a contraceptive diaphragm. These (women) draw a little circle with their fingers at the location of the solar plexus to indicate where they believe the diaphragm to be.

The diaphragm is responsible for about three-quarters of the muscular work of breathing, but, like the beating of the heart, you are not required to feel the work (would we ever *sleep* if we had to feel the work of the heart and the diaphragm?!), so don't go looking for it. You are far better off to go looking for the movement of breathing than the work of breathing. The movement of breathing can be clearly felt. It is a great pleasure to feel the movement of breathing, and there is a world of learning in it.

As the lungs fill with air the diaphragm descends, that is, it goes from a more domed position to a less domed position. It flattens somewhat. As it does so the dimensions of the thorax expand and the diaphragm pushes down on all the viscera between it and the pelvic floor. The whole abdominal wall, from the sternum to the pubis and from the floating ribs to the crest of the pelvis is pushed outward. This expansion of the abdominal and pelvic cavities can be clearly felt, as can the pressure downward on the pelvic floor. If you are tensing, though, sensation will be diminished.

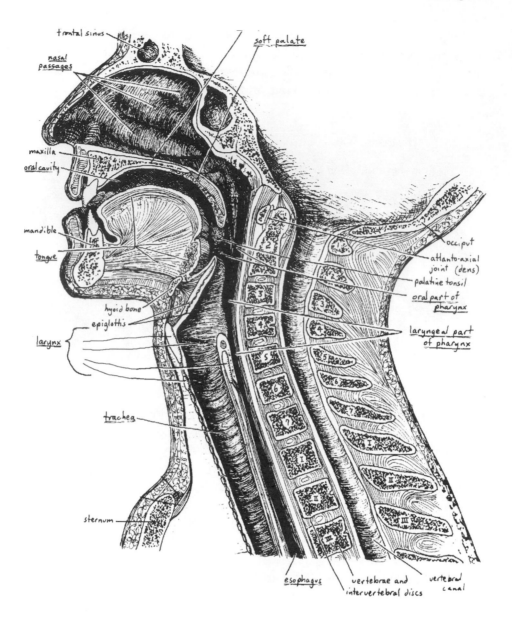

Here are the passageways through which air moves in and out of the body. On the way to the lungs air is warmed and cleaned, especially if it comes into the lungs through the nose. The pharynx goes from the nasal cavity to the trachea. The pharynx is the passageway for both air and (in its oral and laryngeal sections) food. The pharynx is shortened, narrowed, and distorted when the neck muscles tighten. It is easy to see why from this picture. The pharynx is just forward of the weight-bearing (head-bearing) cervical spine. When the cervical vertebrae are jammed they distort the pharynx; at the same time the tongue bunches and invades from the front. What a bind! It is also easy to see how jamming the spine would depress the larynx. Notice all the space for resonance. This is unique to humans, so we can make such lovely sounds. Our purpose with the Technique is to restore that space.

Some implications: it is possible to have a free neck and a long, easy body and still have a tight throat. Some people who are otherwise quite free have chronically tight throats, sometimes because of breathing exercises. If people have done breathing exercises in which they are required to display an audible breath they may come to assume that breath should be audible, to others when doing exercises and to oneself when breathing ordinarily. They make the desired noise by tightening the throat, that is, by tightening the muscles of the pharynx. You can feel those muscles working by swallowing. Notice the condition of them when you finish swallowing. Do you let them be, or do you keep some constriction in them?

It is not possible to have a free throat and a tight neck. If you suffer from a tight throat the culprit is probably your neck. As your teacher helps you free your neck and thereby recover the freedom throughout your body you will be able to free your throat. Singers, wind players, and actors who gasp on inhalation sometimes go on tightening their throats even after tightening is no longer absolutely dictated by general tension. They gradually learn to free neck and throat together.

Likewise the tongue. As the neck frees the tongue can relax. Not before.

When neck muscles tighten all the muscles that surround the lungs tighten, too, in proportion. These are large movement muscles and have no function in breathing, though when things are right with the upper torso those muscles get a round-the-clock massage from the movement of the ribs underneath, which helps to keep them supple. In any case, when the muscles that lie between the ribs and the skin tighten they restrict the mobility of the ribs around the lungs and thereby limit their capacity. A breather who has suffered a limitation in capacity because of downward pull can expect another liter or two of air when he is free from downward pull, because then the ribs can move.

Here we must be clear about what we mean by rib movement. I do not mean a movement of the rib cage, which is a spinal movement. Try it now. Lift your rib cage. That was a movement of your thoracic spine. The rib cage moves as a whole when you do that because it is jointed to the spine. The rib cage moves when the spine moves the same way a hand moves when we bend at the elbow. It's attached so it has to go along. Drop your rib cage. Same thing. Tip it to the side. Same thing, a movement of the spine. See? When I say we must free rib mobility to get air I do not mean movement of the rib cage.

Movement of the rib cage at the spine has no effect on lung capacity. If it did, I don't know how singers would do opera. I have seen every possible position of a rib cage in opera, including recently, hanging backward over the edge of a bed. No, I am talking about the movement of individual ribs at their joints with the vertebrae. Please look at the picture of the lungs as seen from the back. Note that each rib meets a vertebra at an actual joint. What's a joint? Where bones meet so there can be movement. Why do we need so many joints there when we have so few overall? So the ribs can move up and out as the lungs fill, and down and in as the lungs empty. You can feel that movement from the inside and from the outside. To feel it from the outside place your right hand under the shoulder joint of your right arm and then place your left hand flat on your upper chest on the right side with your index finger lying along your collarbone. If you are not pulling down, you will be able to feel the upper ribs moving up and down under your hands. It is the freezing of that movement that limits air capacity.

We need to make another very important distinction here. By rib movement I also do not mean the moving up and down of the sternum. Sternum movement up and down is, like movement of the rib cage, really a movement of the spine. Put your hand on your own sternum and pump it up and down until you really understand. Feel the movement in your spine? So what's the issue?

This is easy to demonstrate and hard to describe, so bear with me. When there is no downward pull in the body the ribs move freely at their joints, bucket-handle fashion, and there is no gross movement up and down of the sternum. The sternum is a quiet but lively (not fixed) island in a rocking sea. But when the upper torso is contracted into downward pull there gets to be a compensatory heaving of the sternum. That's not good. It is an indicator of tension. But if you inhibit the heaving without releasing the downward pull you limit capacity even more than it already is, because you have removed the compensation. This leaves breathers with an enraging frustration. They don't have natural breathing and they also don't have nature's compensation for the loss of it.

By upper rib movement I also do not mean shoulder movement. The arm structure, which includes the collarbone and the shoulder blade, is slung yoke-like over the ribs. The shoulder blade has quite an extension out to the joint with the upper arm to keep the joint quite far up and out in relation to the ribs. That's to allow the ribs to move a lot without interference from arms. That's what we see in the freest singing. The arm structure floats about the ribs and the ribs move bellows-like. What prevents that floating? Downward pull. The contracting of upper torso muscles in downward pull brings the arm structure caving down onto the upper ribs, and it becomes impossible to move the ribs independent of the movement of the clavicle. Another catch-22. If you take a biggish breath you force the clavicle up, which isn't exactly effortless; if you don't force the clavicle up you don't get air. When a student in this bind is told to get enough air but don't move the clavicle he nearly goes mad. If you're his teacher leave him alone until he gets enough freedom that it's a moot point.

Many readers of these last paragraphs will have had to do some pretty radical work on their own maps in order to understand what was said. Many of you when you think of ribs think only of lower ribs. Many singers walk around with their hands on their lower four or five ribs and come to think that's all there are. Since almost nothing can be told about breathing from feeling one's lower ribs, the singers' attention is diverted from the air-ea that matters, the ribs surrounding the lungs. Get to know all your ribs. One student of mine named hers—Miranda, Sarah, Josephine—and traced them with her fingertips before she fell asleep at night. She came to understand that ribs are as individual as fingers, though not as independent. Come to really understand how ribs move so that you can move them as completely and freely as possible. Work with a partner, if you can, who is also learning the Technique. Stand behind your partner and slip you hands gently onto the upper ribs just under the shoulder joint. Ask your partner to breath easily and feel the movement of the upper ribs. Notice how much movement there is at the sides and back. Ask your partner to pull down and notice how the rib movement is restricted. Ask your partner to Alexander up out of the downward pull and notice how the rib movement is freed. If your partner is quite free from downward pull you will feel a wonderful thing at the end of a large breath. There is a keen sensation of the rotation of the upper ribs which the singer feels most clearly with the very top ribs, the ones you can't reach with your hands because of the arm bones. There is a magic in that last bit of rotation which gives a lift to the whole system. One singer said, "When it feels like the upper ribs will take wing and fly you've got it right."

On the subject of air, teachers of breathing tell me they enjoy far more success with their students when they are very clear in their language, particularly when they distinguish air and breath. Air is a substance which occupies the planet along with us. Breath is a reflexive human movement that allows us to move air in and out of our bodies, and the air goes only into our lungs through a short passage. When students understand that air goes only into the upper third of their torsos they are careful to stay free there and awake. Then they are much more likely to allow free breath—that is, movement—throughout their whole torsos. Some students come to me actually believing they must get air into their middle or lower torsos and they do some very strange distorting of the breath as a result, interrupting its wavelike character. The worst consequence of this distortion is the freezing of the upper torso, the very place where freedom counts most. And the happiest consequence of knowing that breath is movement is that it is experienced as movement. More than one student has burst into tears the first time he experienced a simple, sufficient, efficient, reflexive breath.

Breathing Is Movement

Breathing is movement which can be clearly (and deliciously) felt. Free breathing is beautiful to feel and beautiful to see. When we Alexander teachers work with students in supine position we enjoy seeing the movement of breathing organize. Over time as the body frees the breathing releases so that it's like watching waves coming up on a beach. Movement sweeps across the whole torso. The ribs move up and out as the lungs fill and the diaphragm descends, moving the viscera outward against the flexible container. Then the ribs move down and in as the lungs empty and the diaphragm ascends, allowing the viscera to return. There is a quality of repose in this movement when a person is resting on a table which changes to something more dynamic when a person stands and moves into activity. In running the movement of breathing can be dramatic (turn on your TV and watch basketball players who have been playing for a while). In singing the breathing can be both dramatic and reposeful, singing being an interesting instance of taking large amounts of air dictated by something other than an aerobic requirement.

Singing is also an interesting instance of conscious breathing. Singers get very skilled at taking in just the amount of air they will need for a phrase. This requires some degree of intention. Once in a while I meet someone who thinks it's unnatural to bring consciousness to breathing or to regulate the intake of air in any way. I don't think so. I don't know anyone who would advocate always being conscious of breathing or always regulating intake but it's a perfectly natural thing to do for certain purposes, like singing, and people who have a high degree of kinesthetic sensitivity are pleasantly aware of the movement of breathing some of the time or most of the time.

Support for Breathing

The longer I work with breathing the more sources of support for breathing I find. Because most of what passes for support for breathing constitutes instead gross interference, we had better begin by defining our terms. Of the sixteen definitions of support in my dictionary, only two pertain to breathing: 1) to bear or hold up, a structure, mass, part, etc.; 2) to uphold by aid, back up, second. These two definitions are sweetly simple and supremely useful.

Ponder definition number one. *Support*: to bear or hold up, a structure, mass, part, etc. This definition makes a clear distinction between what is supported and what is supporting. As applied to breathing: if we are talking about mass, the breather is supported at the floor; if we are talking about structure, the breathing torso is supported by the legs; if we are talking about a part, the thorax is supported by the lumbar spine. Are there other candidates? Not that I can think of. This definition refers to mechanical support, and the importance of mechanical support in breathing cannot be overestimated. Singers and actors and public speakers who have pulled down and lost their sense of contact with the floor are truly handicapped. Sometimes they don't know how much until they are grounded again. Similarly, if the torso is pulled back and down off the legs by downward pull or mismapping of the pelvis then the legs are not truly felt. Weight is not perceived as balancing on legs; people feel like an unbalanced mass. When this condition is rectified, people say, "It's so wonderful to have *legs* to support me," and it is wonderful. A person can give a speech and all the time she is speaking be enjoying the support of her legs and the security of the floor. Singers who hike their breastbones pull themselves off the supporting lumbar structure and are therefore most likely to invent imaginary support-like strings attached to the breastbone. Don't they wish. When they allow the thorax to settle onto its lumbar support everything gets easy.

Ponder definition number two. *Support*: to uphold by aid, back up, second. Again, we have a basic important distinction, the supporter and the supported. The breathing structures should be left alone to breathe without interference. To attempt to support breathing with breathing structures is ludicrous. Ribs don't support breathing; ribs breathe. The diaphragm doesn't support breathing; it breathes. There are structures and functions that can aid, back up, or second breathing. If the ribs or the diaphragm don't move, you are not breathing and you will die. If the support structures and functions are not moving then breathing won't be glorious but you may still be inhaling and exhaling and you won't die.

So what are the structures and functions that can truly aid or back up breathing? The prime one is your primary control. Your torso may be "moving into length" as you exhale. (I never heard anyone anywhere talk about support for inhaling. There is a felt need for support when we are speaking or singing, which, of course, we do on exhalation.) This "moving into length" can be observed in fine singers and actors and public speakers. It's slight but quite discernible when you get it identified. Its opposite is also visible. Many speakers can be observed to shorten as they exhale. Your teacher will help you learn to coordinate your primary control with your exhaling. When the primary control is fully available for exhalation there is no felt need for effort, and the (necessary) work of controlling the air "stream" is 1) coordinated, 2) natural, that is, it emerges rather than being imposed, and 3) it is sufficient; it gets the job done. The primary control is a function, not a structure, and it is dynamite support. So is the reflex which gives us a sense of a spring in the step. It is activated in the leg when the ball of the foot spreads. I often wondered why certain singers would drop into the ball of the foot at the ends of long phrases. Once I learned about the spring-in-the-step reflex I knew the answer. It's aid for breathing.

How much the resiliency of the abdominal wall actually aids exhaling I don't know, but it certainly aids in the return of the viscera to the pre-inhaling condition. Resiliency depends on 1) being at full stature; in downward pull the abdominals go flabby; 2) not shortening on exhalation, as in any attempt to squeeze air out; 3) not tightening them; tightening abdominals is almost as destructive to exhaling as it is to inhaling; 4) their general tone and strength. Should you do exercises to enhance the strength of the abdominals? Sure, if you want to. It won't help you if you're pulling down, but if you aren't pulling down it's another little oomph. Besides, it feels good. An aside: If you have ever done the pushing-the-stomach-out-for-support thing you will have experienced that it doesn't work. How could it? If you are habituated to it you will have to let it go before you will experience real support.

Everything I have said about the abdominals applies to the pelvic floor. On inhalation the pelvic floor has pressure put on it as the diaphragm descends, pushing the viscera downward and outward. If the pressure is not resisted with tension, then those muscles have a tendency to spring back as the pressure is taken off in exhalation. The springing back feels good. It is certainly experienced as support, and certainly a tensing against it is felt as a loss of support. Here are two views of the pelvic floor.

Musculature of the pelvic floor: adult female, seen from above

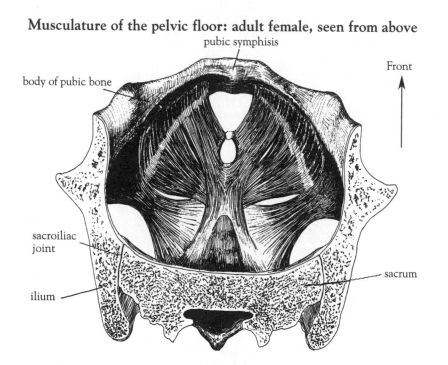

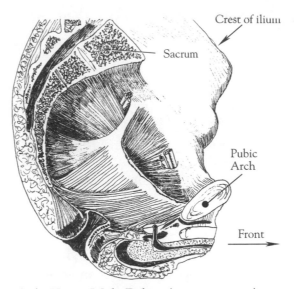

Side View: Male Pelvis (cross section)

And, finally, when the spine lengthens on exhalation there is a pleasant activation of the deep lateral muscles of the pelvis, some fibers of which are continuous with the diaphragm. We feel the lengthening throughout the whole torso when there is no tensing against it, as there is in people who keep these deep muscles in chronic contraction, preventing their recruitment to

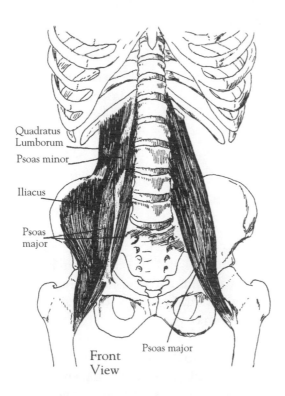

provide support for singing, speaking or wind-instrument playing. My intuition tells me there is another factor in the wonderful feeling that comes in singing when the deep pelvis is truly engaged: the connective tissue. We have five times more connective tissue in the pelvis than any other vertebrate because of the demand for stabilization in radical uprightness. I have the sense that it helps us in breathing, too.

IX. Alexander and the Art of Speaking

Speaking is movement. All the rules that apply to other movement apply as well to speaking. If it is obvious to you that speaking is movement then you probably already speak very well. Most people, however, do not think of speaking as movement. When I say the words, "Speaking is movement," from most people I get an answering blank stare and then a look of recognition as they make a category shift in their minds, "Well, yes, of course, it is, isn't it." When speaking is shifted squarely into the movement category people generally feel relief. If speaking is movement then it is knowable. If speaking is movement then it can be perceived and monitored kinesthetically as one would monitor any other movement for ease and efficiency. Perceiving speaking as movement takes the mystery out of it and eventually takes the effort out of it.

Another useful perspective on speaking is the knowledge that speaking evolved, remarkably. Homo Habilis apparently still had an ape's vocal structure. Homo Erectus showed the beginnings of the arching of the palate but none of the other changes that were necessary to go beyond protospeech. Homo Neanderthalensis had probably advanced sufficiently to speak, but not clearly and not rapidly. Only about one hundred thousand years ago when thoroughly modern Homo Sapiens began to walk the earth was speech as we know it possible. The arching of the roof of the mouth was complete and the voice box had descended to give the throat the requisite shape and length for speaking. The tongue had become more mobile, and an area of the neocortex called Broca's area, not found in nonhuman primates, developed to coordinate speech. Most books will tell you that this vital area coordinates face, tongue, palate, and larynx, but if you read more detailed accounts of the workings of the brain you will learn that the coordination is more complex and more significant, linking conceptualizing and categorizing processes to motor processes. The equipment and the coordination are now there for us to speak very clearly and very rapidly.

Our purpose with the Alexander Technique is to remove interference from the working of our sterling equipment and coordination. To that end we remove first the interference of the downward pull and also the interference of inaccurate body mapping. Then we want to eliminate the interference that comes from mistaken notions about what we are doing when we speak. The most destructive notion I know of is the notion of projection.

It must happen somewhere in the country every night at least once. An actor speaks. A director yells, "Project." The actor tightens his body and speaks louder. The director yells, "Project." The actor tightens even more and speaks even louder and has all sorts of fantasies about where he is sending his voice. He is heard even less well because the tightening has muddied his articulation and thinned his vowels. The director gives up. The actor is discouraged. His problem is the damned word *project* and all the tension-inducing fantasies it generates. Look at the fact: speech and singing are movement, and most of the movement isn't yours. Most of the movement is the air's.

Think about what really happens. Vibrating air is amplified in the resonating cavities and shaped by the articulators. The vibrating of air continues outside you. As vibration moves through water when we drop a pebble in it, so does vibration move through air, in all directions, at a given speed until it dissipates. When the vibration hits the eardrum of a member of an audience it sets the eardrum vibrating, which, with all that happens in the brain, we call hearing.

It should be clear from this description that there is nothing to project. You can project spit, or you can project a spitwad, but you can't project sound, because it isn't a thing. It isn't even a substance. There is not one thing you can do to influence how air vibrates between you and your hearer. It has its own ways.

It is not your business as a speaker to project sound. It is your business to make sound, which is to say, it is your business to set air vibrating just right, and that can only be done inside you. Then the air will vibrate just right all the way to your director's eardrum and he will say, "Thank you very much."

Watch the great actors and the great singers and you will see that they stand there in all their glory and all their simplicity and they produce vibrations in air. They take no responsibility for them beyond producing them. They know that air will continue to do what air has always done. It will vibrate. You will see in these great ones none of the effort associated with the attempt to do something with the sound once it has left them. It is baseball pitchers that are the world's projectors. Not speakers. Not singers.

Do an experiment. The next time someone yells, "Project," inhibit all impulse to obey. Instead lengthen and free and produce the clearest, richest, most simply articulated vibrations you can. I promise you success, and "Thank you very much."

The second most destructive notion people entertain about speaking is a redefining—or an over-defining?—of articulation. The dictionary definition of articulation is "the adjustments and movements of speech organs involved in pronouncing a particular sound, taken as a whole." In other words, articulation is the movement of speaking. But many people think of articulation as an added effort which makes speech clear(er) or tonier or somehow more acceptable. The same director who shouts "Project!" is likely sometime later to shout "Articulate!" If the actor is speaking English sentences she is already articulating, but she may not know that. She may have the notion, like the director, that an added effort in speaking will make her heard. In response to the injunction "Articulate!" the actor will do a tensing similar to what her fellow actor did in response to "Project."

Articulating a sound is simply making it. I advocate taking some time each day, perhaps as you drive in your car or take your shower or do your dishes, to simply articulate consonants and vowels and feel what work is necessary for each sound. You may have so much generalized tension that each phoneme feels pretty much the same. If so, just patiently keep playing with sounds until you begin to sort them out. If you need detailed descriptions of the articulation of particular sounds you can find them in your library.

The question arises, "How much detail does a person need in the map of any part of the body?" It depends. There should be no mismapping. Mismapping always interferes with freedom. An example is the lips. Many people attempt to articulate sound with the lips they put lipstick on. When they form an /m/ or a /b/ they are attempting to form the sounds with a portion of the lips. The speaking lips are larger than the lipstick lips, going all the way to the base of the nose and halfway down to the chin. It is easy to say /m/ or /b/ with the speaking lips, very hard with the lipstick lips.

Some people who want a good working voice for teaching or conversation or singing in a choir will do well to devote an evening or two to getting a general sense of the vocal equipment, the nasal cavity, the oral cavity, and the pharynx, the larynx, and the tongue. People usually find the equipment interesting, and people usually come away from reading about the throat with some added care in the way they eat, given what they learn about human susceptibility to choking.

Persons who earn their livings with their voices and who are devoted to perfecting their crafts may want to cultivate a very detailed and refined map of the areas of vocal production. I know singers who have a high degree of conscious and detailed control over those areas; they are capable of making real choices about their use of those areas. We should not think this is strange or ill-conceived. We are not surprised when a cellist has a highly refined map of her hands and can make choices about how she uses them. The only difference between fingers and tongues and throats and lips is that we can see the fingers and we all use them more or less consciously. The vocal areas are not very available to vision, but they are as available as fingers to our kinesthesia.

People often inquire whether the Alexander Technique is beneficial in returning the vocal cords themselves to health if they are injured. The answer is yes. When generalized misuse is corrected the cords often return to normal. Sometimes Alexander teachers work as part of a team of helpers, a physician, a voice therapist, and an Alexander teacher. This can be a saving combination, especially when the teacher can help the student do the exercises given by the therapist with increasing ease and efficiency.

X. While You're at It, Map Your Brain

To reiterate, a body map may be as complex as you need or as you like. The more accurate your body map is, the freer and more appropriate your moving will be. The more detailed your body map is, the richer your experience of embodiment will be. For purposes of learning the Alexander Technique we give particular attention to mapping the sources of mechanical advantage and of reflex support for voluntary movement. If we want to go on to map the source of constructive conscious control, we must look to the brain, for it is the structure of the brain which accounts for consciousness and for regulation.

Size is not the brain's most astonishing feature, but it is likely to be the one that is remarked. Human brains weigh three and a quarter pounds, in comparison to chimpanzees' twelve ounces, australopithecines' thirteen to eighteen ounces, Homo habilis's twenty-one ounces, Homo erectus's thirty-five ounces. The tremendous evolutionary advantage of more than fifty-two ounces included speech and consciousness, or, to put it another way, categorization and self-knowledge, self-reflection, and self-correction.

Connectivity is the brain's most astonishing feature. The ten billion neurons of the cerebral cortex alone achieve one million billion [sic] connections. All the varied neurons of the brain (one million million [sic]) participate in sweeping, complex, overlapping electrical and chemical patterns across the brain and within areas of the brain. In development, maps are formed which increasingly organize and inform the senses; we use many visual maps when we drive a car, without which visual experience would be chaos and driving impossible. When I first heard Bill Conable talking about body maps I assumed map was a metaphor, but it's not so. Creatures quite literally map sensory territory, and it is another function of brain connectivity which makes it possible to correct the map. Much of our huge brain is up to the business of dealing with itself, which activity is what we experience as self-knowing. We are categories to ourselves and we may, within limits, change ourselves. Alexander's assertion that his Technique provided the next step in evolution failed (so far) because it was framed as a now discredited social Darwinism. It would have fared better as plain old Darwinism. If it was an advance to have such a brain, imagine what an advance it will be to use it! We are surely using our brains when we indulge in constructive conscious control and using the brain for self-regulation is not unnatural in the least. Constructive conscious control is using state-of-the-art equipment according to its design. The brain is designed for self-knowing and self-change.

XI. Common Mapping Errors

You may find as you examine your own body map that you have been operating on some very strange kinesthetic illusions, and you may learn how damaging those illusions have been to free movement. The point here is to remove those illusions forever so that you can recover your primary control. Recovering primary control is easy with an accurate body map, very difficult or impossible without.

This chapter lists some of the common mapping errors that our students have discovered in themselves and some of the consequences of those errors, also what conditions are alleviated when the map is corrected. As you read about other's mapping errors see to what degree you share them. Change your map and note carefully the change in movement.

Many students come with many of these errors in their map, not just a few. For those students correcting the map will result in stunning, fundamental change in body experience and the quality of movement. The improvement is proportional to the error.

For those readers who are studio teachers learning to recognize mapping errors in their students I have tried to indicate some identifying features of the error. Be patient with yourself, remain observant, ask lots of questions of your students, and keeping giving your students sound information, and you will soon be using the mapping material skillfully and effectively.

Some of this material is presented in other chapters, especially Chapter VII. We thought it would be valuable to present it all together here.

THE HEAD:

— that it includes the jaw and begins at the bottom of the jaw. People who believe this will try to move their heads as if from the middle of the neck, four or five vertebrae down from the actual joint. These people almost never look up, as if at the moon, because the scrunching hurts too much, and they can't look down freely down from the head's joint with the spine so they thrust their heads and necks down and forward as a unit if they want to look at a desk. This puts terrible pressure on the area where the cervical curve gives way to the thoracic curve, leading eventually to a painful hump in that area.

— that the base of the skull is a membrane or that the base of the brain is protected only by the top vertebra. One woman told me that every time she moved her head forward and up she imagined that her brain was dripping down her back. Other people tell me they are afraid something will be able to puncture their brains if they leave the area just under the base of the skull unprotected. Needless to say, these people will pull back down again the minute they feel they can in order to prevent the horror the map dictates if they keep going forward and up with their heads. Once they see for themselves that the base of the skull is a very secure, wonderfully protective bony plain they no longer feel the desperate need to pull back down and they begin to learn about freedom.

— that the head moves from the top. These are the people affected by the string-from-the-top-of-the-head fantasy. I devise ingenious little purgatories for teachers who propagate such nonsense. People who try to move their heads from the top always stiffen their necks. When people find out they can move their heads at its bottom at an actual joint they are greatly relieved and they free their necks rather than stiffen them.

— that the head rests on the spine near the back of the base of the skull. Whew! Think of the muscular effort it would take to hold it up! Actually the head *was* supported near its back in ancestral primates. It took nearly ten times the muscle mass to hold the head erect and those creatures weren't even trying to stand upright.

The Neck:

— that it is donut shaped, a sort of O-ring. In one version of this fantasy the muscles of the neck go round and round, a kind of collar. "I feel as though I'm being choked by my neck."

— that the muscles are small and weak.

— that the neck is just at the back. No. The neck includes all the head moving muscles on the front and sides as well as the back. Thinking just of the back of the neck accounts for the weird tucking of the chin that some people do in the attempt to go forward and up with their heads, freeing the back of the neck (so they think) at the expense of the front. This is especially common in Europe where Alexander's word *neck* is sometimes translated into a German word that does mean the back of the neck. Tricky.

— that the bottom of the neck is at the top of the collar, especially common in men. The poor men drop everything south of the top of the collar into the chest in their maps and suffer a caving-in of the top of the torso as a result. Usually the buttons on a button-down shirt fall right at the collarbone, so if you must map your body with regard to your clothes (not a good idea) then please map your neck at the bottom of your business collar, not at the top.

COMMON ERRORS

— that the muscles of the neck surround one or two or three vertebrae. No. They surround seven vertebrae. They do also on a giraffe. The giraffe just happens to have foot-deep vertebrae. When people get nicely lengthened out and they say they feel like a giraffe, they are getting closer to the truth. They are like a giraffe.

— that the neck muscles have some role in speaking and singing. Not here on earth. In heaven there are great choirs of neck muscles finally getting to sing, but not here. The neck muscles only get to move the head around to look here and there as the singer sings, here at the lover, there at the moon, there at the surprising letter just brought by the footman, there at the floor, back at the lover, back at the moon, and so on and so on.

THE TONGUE:

— that it originates somewhere near the back of the mouth, usually just beneath the back of the hard palate. Try it. Just try moving your tongue from there. Impossible. It makes me want to scream when I try it, yet singing students and acting students coast to coast are earnestly trying to move and free their tongues from there. When they discover the truth that the tongue originates in the throat just above the hyoid bone, and then makes its way up and over into the jaw, and is therefore long, long, long, suddenly freeing it becomes possible.

— that the tongue is moved by muscles in the throat. Yipes! Actually the tongue is one of the few instances in the body where a muscle's moving itself is the point, not a muscle's moving bone. Actually the tongue is a composite muscle—like a composite flower!—more than forty muscles in one neat little package. That's why it can go all over the place.

THE LIPS:

— that the lips that form consonants are the lips we put lipstick on. The moving, consonant-forming lips are much bigger, going all the way up to the base of the nose and all the way down to the base of the gum. Have a look at the facial muscles again and play with moving the movement lips. The lipstick lips just ride along.

THE FACE:

— that the face is skin on bone, a ruinous fantasy for an actor or a singer, often deriving from the word *mask* as applied to the face. Imagine the little purgatory I have devised for the monster who developed the face-as-mask notion.

COMMON ERRORS

— that lifting the cheeks contributes to resonance. This fantasy accounts for the look of perpetual astonishment often seen in aspiring opera singers. It's a dramatically disastrous notion. It doesn't work, of course, because it means that the facial muscles are not available for what they are intended for, dramatic expression. Facial expressions of joy, despair, and cruelty are forever lost to the singer who feels compelled to keep the cheeks hiked.

THE THROAT:

— that the esophagus (the swallowing tube) is in front of the trachea (the breathing tube). It's *behind* it. (See page 70.) This common confusion makes swallowing much more laborious and tightens the voice as we try to act out our maps.

THE JAW:

— that it hinges behind the ear. Try out what this would be like.

— that it hinges at the two ends of the horseshoe shape at the bottom. Try it.

— that it hinges just below the corners of the mouth. (Jaw=chin.) Try it.

— that there is bone filling in the whole horseshoe at the bottom. Try it.

— that its joint is at the coronoid process, the roughly triangular projection which slides along the cheekbone as the jaw opens. Try it.

— that there are two jaws, an upper and a lower. Try it.

THE LUNGS:

— that the lungs are in the abdominal cavity. Persons who believe this put their hands on the lower ribs to try to monitor the amount and flow of air.

— that the lungs are in the pelvic cavity. These persons put their hands on their bellies to feel air. Of course, what they are feeling is the movement of the viscera forward as the diaphragm descends.

— This might as well go here as anywhere: some people have an *air column* in their maps, sometimes of monstrous length. If you hear your student mention his air column ask him to draw it. You'll be astounded by what you see. Show the student just exactly what does occupy that space in his body and he'll be grateful to you forever.

— that lungs are hideously vulnerable to puncture and must therefore be protected by tightening muscle around them. Actually they are protected by the ribs and the two shoulder blades lying directly over them like medieval shields. Besides, tightened muscles are themselves quite puncturable.

THE DIAPHRAGM:

— that it is a vertical structure, perhaps the top of the abdominal muscles. People tighten abdominal muscles to conform to this fantasy and thereby destroy in the movement of breathing the tide of the gut forward as the diaphragm descends. The diaphragm is a dome-shaped muscle which separates the thoracic cavity from the abdominal cavity, horizontally.

— that it is in the abdominal cavity.

— that it is in the pelvic cavity. The muscles at the very bottom of the pelvis which support the abdominal contents are sometimes called the *pelvic diaphragm*. They are important, too, but they have non-metaphorical individual names and are not the same as the *thoracic*, or respiratory diaphragm.

THE RIBS:

— that there are six or eight of them and that they surround the abdominal cavity. This fantasy leaves people feeling terribly vulnerable in their upper bodies. People feel so much safer when they learn that their ribs come all the way up to the bottom of their necks, that they surround the whole thoracic cavity as well as some of the abdominal cavity, that they even underlie the shoulder blade, the shoulder joint, and the breasts, that they provide the first line of defense against lung puncture by entirely surrounding both lungs and heart (which nestles between the lungs).

— that there is a rib *cage*. Cage is a terrible metaphor for ribs. The bars of a cage are fixed so that what's inside can't get out. Imagine you visit the zoo. The zoo keeper says to you, "We're so proud of the lion cage. It has a clever arrangement whereby the top of the bars are made of cartilage so that they're nice and springy and the bottom of the bars are jointed with the floor so that plenty of movement is possible."

— that upper ribs shouldn't move in breathing. This fantasy destroys singers.

— that ribs are only in front; the back is something (vague and) different.

— Women often believe that they have breast tissue interior to the ribs, crowding the lungs. Some believe that there are no ribs underneath their breasts, and many fail to clearly perceive the rib area above their breasts. Consequently they stop the natural movement of upper ribs, and their breathing suffers.

COMMON ERRORS

COMMON ERRORS

— that ribs expand, maybe like rubber bands or a telescope, or by coming right out of their joints! Actually, the volume of the thoracic cavity expands when the ribs are lifted from the sides. They pivot at the front cartilage and at the spine, rather like the handle of a bucket. Check this on yourself; there is a good picture of it in the *Anatomy Coloring Book*.

— that the front of the ribs or the sternum lines up with the lumbar spine.

THE BACK:

— that the back is the body's main support, rather than the spine.

— that the spine is just the little bumps you can feel running down your back.

— that the back is some sort of solid bony plate.

THE SPINE:

— that it is small, as big around as a dime, or a quarter, or a fifty-cent piece.

— that it is a rod, "like a broom handle."

— that it bears weight near the surface of the back.

— that the weight-bearing part of it is exterior to the ribs.

— that it is straight. Some people do manage to make it nearly so.

THE PELVIS:

— that the pelvis is a bowl. The pelvis is so little like a bowl it won't even hold a ten pound baby once nature has decided it's time for the baby to leave its mother's womb. The pelvis of a full-size skeleton might hold a soccer ball if the pelvis were never tipped because the pubic bone does come up some in front, but it wouldn't begin to hold a bunch of soft balls and it certainly won't contain strawberries and cream.

— derived from the bowl image, perhaps, that the pelvis covers the abdomen in front.

— that there are spool-shaped "sits bones" or "sit bones" appended to the bottom of the pelvis on which we must precariously balance. Rather, the pelvis itself is rocker-shaped at the bottom, providing a support that is reliable in any position.

— that the pelvis is one massive bone, therefore vulnerable. Rather the pelvis is two medium-sized bones jointed at the pubis to each other, at the top to the sacrum (the delta-shaped bone at the bottom of the spine) on either side, and near the bottom to the thigh bone on either side. There is considerable ability to bear impact because of the cushioning at the pubic symphysis (not a bone, but the place where the two pubic bones meet) and some resilience at the sacroiliac joints, and then, of course, it's nicely padded all around.

—that the front of the pelvis lines up with the lumbar spine.

— that there is no movement in the pubic and sacroiliac joints. In fact, there is some—a little—with every breath.

The Pelvic Cavity

— that it goes straight down, like a plastic bag or a pillowcase. Actually it opens back at the bottom, as you will see if you look at the pictures on pages 64 and 65. People who unconsciously make the pillowcase assumption try to reshape themselves to match it.

The Pelvic Floor:

— that it is mostly bone with little holes.

The Sacrum:

— that it is part of the pelvis. Not really. It is five fused vertebrae, so its origin is spinal. It delivers weight at its very top sideways into the thickened part of the pelvic bones on either side, where weight is then delivered through the hip joints into the thighbone.

The Tailbone:

— that it must bear the body's weight in sitting or standing. People say, "My tailbone gets so sore because it has to take all my weight. It's so small."

If the tailbone had to take our weight it would soon disappear. Tiny bones disintegrate under lots of weight. Fortunately, in standing our weight is delivered out to the thigh bones, and in sitting it is delivered down into the rockers well in front of the tailbone, which just floats there. I have explained elsewhere that the non-weight bearing part of the sacrum and the tailbone are in the body to shape Levis. (They also form the attachments for important muscles and ligaments.)

COMMON ERRORS

COMMON ERRORS

THE HIP JOINTS:

— that they are near the top of the pelvis, often at the iliac crest. This illusion creates lower back pain and interferes with mobility at the hip joints. It's one of the factors in the phenomenon which in the vernacular is called tight-assed.

— that they are quite close together. Epidemic among dancers, who tend to think of the hip joints as being just on either side of the pubis *inside* the pelvis. That's where ninety percent of them put the tips of their index fingers when they work on turnout. I always imagine the heads of their femurs looking at each other across a little space, never quite able to touch. If this fantasy were true, of course, none of us would have had a human birth.

— that they are a ball and socket, the socket being separate from the pelvis and massive. You should see the drawings. Ball and socket is a bad metaphor.

— that the sockets open toward the floor and the thigh bone is stuck up into it deep in the pelvis. For these people movement of the leg more than a few inches in any direction is ill-advised.

— that it is a joint at which the legs can move in relation to the torso, but not the torso in relation to the legs. These mappers believe that they must bend forward from their waists because it is their only option. The torso just can't move forward at the hip joints. Such a person may take five minutes to begin to figure out how to go into monkey, and movement of the torso forward at the hip joint will at first feel supremely strange and then supremely wonderful. People say, "*That's* what my tennis coach has been trying to get me to do!" You don't want to know what the tennis coach says.

— that it is a line at the very bottom of the torso, like a Raggedy-Ann doll.

— that the legs are attached to the "sit bones" (ischial tuberosities) at the very bottom of the pelvis.

— that the joint is at the top of the arch of the groin, and that the resilient tendon of the gracilis muscle is bone.

— that legs are attached to each other and the genitals lie below the meeting of the two thigh bones.

THE KNEE:

— that the kneecap is the knee, that is, the place where weight is delivered. Drop into downward pull and notice that it feels that way.

— that there is a bone between the thigh bone and the bone(s) of the lower leg called the knee. Most people with their bodies mapped that way will draw the knee as about the size of a baseball, usually round.

— that the joint of the thigh and the lower leg is just behind the kneecap or just above it. When these people learn that it is at the bottom of the kneecap that movement is possible, they suddenly feel that they have luxuriously long thighs.

—that the knee doesn't go all the way round!

THE ANKLE:

— that it is the two bumps that are the bottom of the leg bones. People really try to swivel the foot from those two points. In my old map those bumps were the top of two bones that went all the way down into the ball of the foot. No wonder it took me many months to recover full range of motion at the ankle *after* I had correctly mapped it.

— that the ankle is at the top of the heel bone in back, in the depression just forward of the Achilles tendon. This is consistent with the L-shaped foot.

— that the ankle is not a joint at all, but just where the leg ends and the foot begins. People who won't release the ankle as they come out of downward pull often fall in this category. They are not moving forward onto the arch of the foot because they don't believe they can.

THE FOOT:

— that the foot is L-shaped, that weight passes down through the back of the lower leg into the back of the heel and forward into the rest of the foot.

— that the toes are part of the arch, causing a gripping of the toes.

THE SHOULDER:

— that there is one upper arm joint instead of two. Suffice it to say this error often ends in injury and always limits technique. The one joint is fantasized as being somewhere between the two actual joints, which are the joint of the collarbone and the sternum and the joint of the upper arm with the shoulder blade.

— deriving from the above-stated error, that the upper torso is relatively or completely immobile. The person who does not know that there is a joint of the collarbone and sternum from which movement up and down and back and forward is available will never make those movements, even when it makes perfect sense to, as in swimming. When they begin to move there because someone show them that the joint exists, they are first incredulous and then delighted because movement there feels so good.

— also from the same source, that the shoulder blades are attached to the spine and therefore not mobile.

— that the shoulder blades are attached to each other and therefore not mobile.

— that the shoulder blades are attached to the ribs and therefore not mobile.

— that the shoulder blades are attached to the base of the skull and therefore not mobile. Actually, this one is rare, but I mention it anyway.

— that the upper arm attaches to the spine, or to a socket off the side of the spine. This usually derives from a teacher's saying something like, "Well, the arms really come off the back," a statement that is defensible on certain grounds but which will profoundly confuse some students if it is not made utterly clear what is meant.

— that the upper arm attaches to the ribs.

— that the upper arm attaches to a socket attached to the base of the skull.

— that there is a shoulder girdle which is a mirror image of the pelvic girdle. In this fantasy most of the upper torso is bone and immobility is dictated by the map.

THE ELBOW:

— that the elbow is the bump at the bottom of the ulna, often mapped as separate from the ulna, usually regarded as capable of slipping and causing all sorts of difficulties.

— that the joint is of *an* upper arm bone and *a* lower arm bone, in which case the lower arm will not be mapped for rotation and the student is likely to do rotating at the joint of the upper arm and shoulder blade that should be done at the elbow instead. (For instance, turning a door handle or a steering wheel.)

— that the lower arm rotates around the radius, that is, around an axis on the thumb side of the lower arm. This error is the cause of most tendinitis at the wrist or elbow in musicians, carpenters, and tennis players.

COMMON ERRORS

THE WRIST:

— that the wrist is those two bumps at the bottom of the radius and ulna.

— that it is the place above those bumps where you wear your wrist watch.

— that the hand bones meet the arm bones directly, creating a hinge effect. People can actually give the wrist a hinge-like character if they believe this.

— that the hand turns over at the wrist and the forearm isn't part of the motion

— that the wrist is a ball and socket

— that the rest position of the hand is the thumb lined up with the radius. This insures a chronic contraction of the outside of the wrist and destroys the inch or inch and a half of mobility at the wrist toward the thumb side of the hand. This is a serious handicap for pianists. They need that inch or so of movement.

THE HAND:

— that the fingers begin at the edge of the palm where the lines are seen that seem to people to correspond to the lines at the first and second joints of the fingers, counting from the tips. In fact those lines fall between the second and third joints, as can be readily seen by looking not at the palm but at the back of the hand. People who try to place the joint at the lines on the palm always have stiff fingers and a curled back of the hand that ruins finger dexterity.

— that fingers have muscles. There are muscles that attach to the finger tendons near the proximal ends of the fingers, but there is no muscle that can be *built* on fingers the way a bicep is built on an upper arm, which is what some people imagine, especially when they do finger exercises.

— that the palm contains no muscles.

— that the bone (!) in the palm is a bony plate like a shoulder blade. Really there are four bones (not counting the thumb) and they move!

— that the thumb is the first two segments from the tip, putting its connection at the edge of the palm, not at the wrist. People who have the thumb mis-mapped have lost significant mobility of the thumb and always have a very prominent second joint and a sort of caved-in space between the second joint and the wrist.

XII. For Teachers: How to Help Your Students with Their Maps

Teachers being the generous souls that they are most often ask this question in workshops, "How can I help my students correct their maps?" Alexander teachers are eager to know how to recognize mapping errors and correct them because they have seen for themselves that it speeds learning the Technique significantly and with some students it makes the difference between success and failure. Teachers of musicians, actors, dancers, and athletes are in some cases desperate to know how to help because they see that it makes such a difference in performance, in many cases the difference between winning or losing. There is the further incentive of wanting to give the student the tools to stay free of pain and injury in the student's future career. Many teachers quite rightly want to help their students stay free of the suffering they themselves have endured. Many are unclear how to do that. What constitutes effective prevention? is a sub-question under What can I do for my students?

This section of this Manual is directed to both Alexander teachers and teachers of artists and athletes. It should have some relevance for teachers of anything.

First, how do you know when to be concerned about a student's map? Simple. When the student is having difficulty learning, or in the case of Alexander teaching, difficulty following the perfectly good direction and guidance you are giving with your hands. When the student cannot free her tongue. When the student can't put his head in relation to the violin without collapsing his chest. When the student can't go up on toe without arching her back. When standard work does not improve the actor's articulation. When the tennis player can't learn to bend at the hip joint to wait for the serve. When the back of Susie's hand continues to curl at the piano no matter what is said, done, demonstrated, coaxed, begged, or threatened.

At the point where the student is having difficulty you have two choices with regard to the map. You can inquire into the student's current map, or you can simply give accurate information based on what you observe. Time available will probably be the deciding factor. If you opt to find out what in the student's current map is causing the incapacity, simply ask, "Tell me how you think about breathing." "What's a wrist like?" "How does a person make facial expression, anyway, do you suppose?" Then wait while your student gains access to what's she's really thinking. If she says, "Well, I guess I never thought about what a wrist is like," then say, "Suppose you think about it now. What's your best guess?" You will eventually get an answer with some specificity, "Well, I think it's a hinge joint." Then go for more detail, "How does it work, exactly. What hinges to what?" "I think the hand hinges to the arm." "How?" "Well, let's see, like a door. I think the hand flaps back and forth like a door." "Show me." She flaps her hand in relation to the arm. "How does the hinge allow for movement side to side?" "I don't think it does, really." "Because it's a hinge." "Yes."

At this point you have concrete information about her map of her wrist. It took only a minute or two to get it and a little patient questioning. Suppose she's a cellist. Suppose you have spent already many hours trying to help her achieve the easy movement at the wrist that characterizes free cello bowing. Nothing has really worked. What do you have to lose by spending a few minutes to see if an accurate map of her wrist will help her? Say to her something like this, "I have good news for you. The wrist isn't after all a hinge. If it were nobody would play a cello, and everyone who thinks it's a hinge has the stiffness you have. The stiffness is completely consistent with the way you think about your wrist. Fortunately a wrist isn't the least bit hinge-like. The wrist is designed for maximum mobility of a hand so that there can be cellists."

Tell your student to spend the next several weeks becoming intimately acquainted with her own wrist. Give her a Xerox of the wrist page of the *Anatomy Coloring Book* and tell her to make ten copies of it. She should put one in her cello case, one in her car, one on the bathroom mirror, one on her bedroom mirror, one on her practice stand, and five in five other places where she will see a wrist many times a day and be reminded of the elegance and adequacy of her own structure.

Notice, teachers, that this is a very small expenditure of time and effort on your part compared to many other choices you have for helping your students solve their problems. Imagery, for instance. Imagery is time consuming and exhausting when applied to movement. The student struggling to imagine a river flowing through her wrist is even less likely to feel what's actually going on there than when she was imageless. The place for images in teaching is after the fact, not before it. When your student has her wrist mapped correctly and is bowing easily and fluidly she may very well say to you, "You know, I just love this feeling. It's like a river is flowing through my wrist and into the bow to the string." You just smile, and say, "Good." You can smile at that point because you understand what has happened. Your student has freed her arm from the tyranny of the mistaken map. That freeing has insured the fluidity of the movement. In the absence of her former tensing she is experiencing an actual flow through her arm, something impossible when she was tensing. Now she uses a lovely image to describe a feeling of freedom. Freedom often produces images; images never produce freedom. Images before the fact is like going to a fine restaurant and eating the menu. Images after the fact is dessert.

Your most important resource in this imaginary exchange with your imaginary cello student was the picture of the wrist. No student will take your word for it if you merely describe the part you hope the student will remap. The map is too powerful. It will win against words, especially for those students who tend to access their own maps visually. Even with skeletons and pictures some students will say, "I really don't think my body is like that." One man had to go to his university library — he was a university professor — and look at thirty or forty different anatomy books before he finally conceded that the lungs are in the upper torso, not the belly. He was so certain he was right. He could feel the air rising through his torso when he sang. What he felt was a tortuous progressive tensing from the bottom of his torso to the top which he created to make it feel like air was rising through his torso as he sang. It's because these map-created feelings are so persuasive internally that you need all the evidence for the truth that you can amass.

So pester your school to get you the visual aids you need. A full-size skeleton is wonderful to have. Music teachers need them far more than they need computers. Tell your department head that you prefer a skeleton to a computer. It'll get you a promotion for good sense.

There is an 18" flexible skeleton available that is very useful* . One piano teacher put her small skeleton at a small grand piano from a toy store on top of her teaching piano. In 30 seconds she could illustrate for the young students just how they should be sitting on the rockers at the bottom of the pelvis, just how they could bend forward at their hip joints, just how they could rock from rocker to rocker to go to the ends of the keyboard, just how they could balance their heads, just how they needed to let the shoulder blades move. There are large laminated charts of the bony structure and musculature that are very helpful and plastic models of everything from your guggle to your zatch. One voice teacher I know uses the model of the vocal mechanism and finds it very helpful.

Young students love to learn about their bodies, and visual aids are particularly important for young students. Little ones comprehend the truth just by there being pictures of the truth everywhere. There are some mapping issues so critical to success with an instrument that I believe they should be addressed at the very beginning, before a child picks up an instrument or puts hands on a keyboard. Some teachers have worked out clever ways of introducing the truth about the rotation of the lower arm in the very first lesson so that the arms always function well and the hand never abandons a happy relationship with the arm. One way is to use a large sheet of cheap paper. Ask the child to place his arm and hand on the paper with his palm up and rapidly draw around it with a pencil. Then ask him to turn his hand over and draw around it again. The fact of the axis will be obvious and the child can rotate his arm back and forth and see just how it works. The drawing looks like a butterfly, and the child can bring his arm off the paper and go on rotating it.

---

* A good source is Anatomical Chart Company, 8221 Kimball Avenue, Skokie, Illinois, 60076, telephone 800-621-7500.

The teacher calls this making butterflies in the air, and she instructs the child to go on making butterflies as he brings his hands to the keyboard for the first time. The little hand and arm are just right and the child will keep them light and easy. The teacher then shows the child how to move the axis around the keyboard and how to allow the hands and lower arms to simply fall within the axis easily to play.

Another way to make this clear is to put a little sun sticker on the bottom of the radius. As the child rotates the arm she can watch the sun go from morning on through noon to sunset, but then she sees that she has to bring the sun back through noon again to go back to morning.

It is easy for the teacher to show the child how much movement there is in the wrist to begin to move to octaves, for instance, or to trill. All the teacher says is, "Look, if you start with your butterfly, you can go all the way toward the little finger and then back or all the way toward the thumb and then back." If the child does not go back to the rest position the teacher can say, "This is a place to go back to your butterfly."

I hope that teachers will find simple, quick ways to help young students to begin their training with accurate maps. Young students love to learn about their structures. They will eagerly absorb anatomy books. One child I saw gets very excited when he see a Skediton as he calls it, and he immediately asks questions about it and spontaneously makes connections to his own body. If every child had such an opportunity so much misery would be prevented.

Watch your Language

I don't have to tell you what happens when you use the *P* word or the *R* word with your students. If you use the *P* word (*posture*) you will get rigidity, and if you use the *R* word (*relax*) you will get collapse. Both conditions are worse than useless for making music. Yet some teachers go on using them year after year, frustrated by the results they get but unclear what to do instead.

Here's what to do instead. Create for yourself a list of body words that work to procure for your students the physical condition that is conducive to playing and singing. Take a dictionary of reasonable size and go through the whole dictionary page by page looking for useful body words. This is not the gigantic task it may sound like. It takes less time than reading a book, and it is fun. Perusing the dictionary is how I found *stature*, a word Alexander used, but I missed it somehow in my reading of Alexander. I didn't understand its profound usefulness. It's the most helpful word to me in my own use. If when I free my neck and lengthen and widen my back I am thinking of coming effortlessly to full stature, I never go wrong.

So create a movement lexicon to use in your teaching, and then watch carefully to see what the result of each word is. Keep a small notebook with comments beside each word describing what you actually saw and heard in your students when you used your movement words. One band director told me the most useful word he had found was comfortable. He had struggled with the *R* word for years, observing that it almost never got good results, so now he is delighted, because he tells me when he says as he brings his baton up, "Okay, band, get your bodies really comfortable to play," the players do exactly that! He even gets feedback from the audience in the very words he used in rehearsal, "Your band always looks so comfortable."

Here are some suggestions, so you get the idea.

comfortable	easy	effortless	effortlessly
balanced	supported	light	free
freedom	stature	buoyant	buoyancy
lighten	feathery	floating	smooth
elegant	graceful	facility	elegance
luxurious	poise	steady	secure
grounded	in contact	stable	stability
balanced	move	movement	mobility
motion	firm	strong	rooted

These are a few. You will find more and you will gradually incorporate into your speaking to students the words that work best for you and them. The important thing here is that you are constantly referring students to their own actual experience in their own actual bodies. You need to be referring them to their own experience at least ten or fifteen times in each teaching hour. "Take an easy, sufficient breath and begin." I guarantee these words will be more effective than "Take a deep breath and begin." "Balance on the bench and begin." "Don't forget to bring the bow up elegantly." "Simply, now; no fuss." "Wide awake in your bodies, please, as we begin." "Alert and easy, y'all." "Whole body, whole world, gang." "My friend, just stop and get your fluidity back. Thanks." "Do it again and let it be grounded this time." "You'll like it better if you sing with a body than without one. Try it again." "That time you really let your body lengthen on the down bow. Good."

This last comment is a little different from the others, which are injunctions, teachers' best friend. The last comment is feedback, naming. If you constantly, quietly, consistently name what your student is doing right (yes, Alexander teachers, there is a right way to go up—the easy way that liberates you) you will be creating a secure base of understanding in them. I am astonished at the number of teachers who only name what they want the student to change. Err, if you must, in the other direction. Only name what you want them to go on doing just as they are. Or name what's useful in what they are doing and invite them to make it more useful, "It's good you're noticing what you are doing with your head and neck. Now expand your awareness to take in the rest of you as you play and you'll really have a useful gestalt." "That's much easier in three arm joints. Now add a fourth, please." "You're doing great with your body awareness. Any chance for some world awareness, too?"

Keep Checking

Keep asking your students how they are doing with each of the mapping changes they are making. Some students incorporate new information quickly. A map can change forever in three days, so after seven days some students will come back into your studio truly changed since their last lesson as a consequence of correcting a mapping error. If you see change just credit it and go on to the next thing. You might say, "I see you have really understood about the movement of your ribs. Good. No more sufficiency of air problems. Now if you can come to understand your lower torso as well as you now understand your upper torso you can get some real support for exhalation."

If, on the other hand, there is little change or no change, it is very important to note that and to discover the reasons for it. "You are still breathing in a way consistent with your old map. How come?" If you find the student has done no internal work on the map, then you say, "Remember that in movement the map always wins. You will go on breathing based on the way you think you are structured, and you will never have enough air nor will you ever know what to do with the air you have. You're going to have to change your map definitively, or there won't be any further improvement in your breathing." Naming the truth so frankly is not always easy, but it's lots easier than going on week after week facing a student who isn't learning.

If your student has made some improvement, name the improvement and inquire. "That's much better breathing than last week, but it won't get you happily through the music you're working on. Tell me what you actually did with the information I gave you last week." You will probably find that your student used the information some of the time but not all the time. Remind the student that consistent intention is important. Say things like, "For the next few weeks it will be very important to keep accessing the truth about your structure so that you can breathe well every time you practice."

There is a discipline in correcting a map where it's been incorrect, but it's a gentle discipline and there is powerful internal reinforcement because what was hard becomes easy and what was murky becomes clear. You will find that you can constantly refer students to their own experience and to their own structures right in the thick of teaching anything.

XIII. If You Exercise

I believe that F.M. Alexander would take a different attitude toward exercise today than he did in his day, when he scorned exercise because he decried the excess effort it commanded and the injuries it caused and the unawareness it fostered. I believe that he would credit the recent research that documents the necessity for aerobic activity (perhaps it could have delayed or prevented his stroke!), and I believe he would have welcomed the increased muscle tone that sophisticated weight training cultivates and the enhanced movement at joints and appreciation of the spine that comes from yoga and t'ai chi. I believe he would have enjoyed seeing people running on our streets and have taken a wry pleasure in the sight of people jazzercising.

I believe Alexander would have acknowledged that students who exercise by today's methods, no matter how badly, learn more quickly than those who don't, because they have come to value movement, if only crudely, and because they have tone in their bodies, even if effort-induced and effort-filled, which offers them a glimmer of insight into what is possible. Movement has inspired in them a hunger for freer movement. They hope that if sport or programmed movement has improved their lives, freer movement might revolutionize their lives. Exercise is a foot in the door of kinesthetic apathy for many students.

Which Exercise? For What?

I ask students in the first lesson or two whether they exercise and, if so, how. I want to show them early in their learning Alexander's principles how those principles apply to what they do. And I want to know what kind of movement the student has come to value. Answers to the question fall into several categories. Some students prize aerobic activity, like swimming or running, that boosts the oxygen economy of their bodies. Some enjoy movement that increases flexibility, like calisthenics. Some like energy-enhancing endeavors, like t'ai chi and yoga. Some have been prescribed exercises by their physical therapists. (These students typically are scared not to perform the exercises for fear they will feel even worse than they do now.) Some students are obsessed with strength and "work out" in order to be or feel stronger. Some care not at all about how they feel, but exercise in order to look a certain way, which some express in strange metaphors like hard or flat.

A special subset of students exercises because it is their job to do so, or so they see it. Athletes stretch and run and strain and dancers do bar work in preparation for what "they really do," play basketball or dance. Pianists, even, will sometimes tell me they do finger exercises in order to strengthen their fingers, as if depressing a piano key were an extraordinary feat requiring prepared muscles. I always question the unexamined premises that justify the expenditure of effort. Sometimes the assumptions are valid —strengthening the muscles with which a basketball player jumps results in a remarkable increase in capacity—and sometimes they are not—piano playing itself develops the strength and dexterity necessary for the task.

In any case, the point is this: those who exercise may have their cake and eat it, too. The same dedication of time and effort can result in two beneficial effects, not one. People may gain aerobic capacity *and* primary control. They may have flexibility *and* primary control. (Actually, flexibility, of all these qualities, is possible only with primary control, as I hope I can prove.) Students may cultivate chi and prana *and* primary control. They may be strong *and* supple.

If Your Exercises are Prescribed for Therapy

Physicians and physical therapists often prescribe exercises for maladies such as tendinitis and aching lower backs and rotator cuff problems in the arms. Sometimes the exercises are carefully chosen and really do address the problem. Other times they are general, printed on a single sheet of paper and handed out like aspirin. Even when the exercises are carefully chosen they are rarely carefully taught, so students bring to the exercises the same misconceptions they bring to other uses of the same structures and with the same result, strain and injury. I remember a violinist who came to me because of the tendinitis in her wrist. She had been given quite rigorous and detailed exercises for her wrist, some of them involving the use of darling little weights. Unfortunately the young woman did the exercises with the same misunderstanding of the rotation of her lower arm and the same retraction across the wrist that she exhibited in violin playing, so she cried each day after she finished her exercises; but she persisted in them because she figured they must be good for her or they wouldn't have been prescribed. When the movement in the exercises was retrained so that it was in keeping with her structure, then it did benefit her. It is important to understand that the exercises given you by your doctor will only help you if you do them well.

You will need to read your instructions carefully so that you understand what is actually being prescribed. Sometimes a careful reading is difficult or impossible because the text is written so badly. You may have to guess, or more often, you may have to translate the language of the instructions into movement language that makes sense. An example: exercise instructions often say such things as, "Bring your chin to your chest," or "Bring your ear toward your shoulder." People who take those instructions at face value often shorten and stiffen their necks as they move to do the exercise and thereby prevent any possibility of its doing what it is designed to do, relieve pressure on the vertebrae of the neck. I ask my students to always translate such language by referring to the joint being used and to the movement being made. So "Bring your chin to your chest," becomes "Allow your head to tilt forward gently at its joint with your spine. Be sure to keep your neck muscles free and be sure the movement incorporates the little movement up that facilitates your primary control in the movement. Be sure the movement has a quality of release."

The pictures that accompany your exercises may be as problematic as the words. A student who was herself a physical therapist brought a booklet of neck exercises to her lesson once. She had been doing the exercises for several weeks for her stiff neck and now her neck was not only stiff but also aching. The booklet was glossy and had color photographs of one of the tensest persons I have ever seen in print illustrating the exercises. My student was imitating what she saw on the page and suffering predictable consequences. If you look at the pictures in your exercise instructions and you see a pulled-down person doing the exercises, do not imitate the pulled-down person. Release instead out of your own downward pull and do the exercises in a way that further releases you. You will know you are on the right track if you end the exercise period feeling more alert and comfortable.

If you are given special equipment by your physical therapist please use it sensibly. My students sometimes bring me the traction apparatus for their necks that features a bag of water to hang over a door for the weight of traction. If a student is attentive and lengthens gently under the pull on their necks it can feel quite good to them. If, on the other hand, the student's response to the weight is to pull down against it the apparatus is harmful rather than beneficial. The rule is: it's not what's done but how it's done.

Alexander and your Aerobic Exercise: Walking and Running

A few of my students got into serious trouble because they did not sufficiently distinguish walking and running. One had taken up speed-walking and had pushed the speed of her walking past the moment when the body goes naturally into running, a moment which the gait labs have shown is relative to our size. Walking when we should be running is a serious strain on the body and always results eventually in pain. Walk fast, by all means, if it feels good to you, but be respectful of that magic moment when the gait just naturally alters. Similarly, be sure you do not jog so slowly that you should be in a fast walk. Sometimes trainers will notice that a trainee's pulse rate in running is above what is safe for the person and advocate slowing down. If slowing down results in the trainee's running when he should be walking he will experience a harmful heaviness in the jogging. If you need to slow down to bring a pulse rate down, then just walk for a while and begin running again when you need to elevate the pulse again.

Be likewise respectful of the length of your stride. It, too, is built into your neurology proportional to your size. If you make it chronically longer or shorter you will suffer in your joints, or if you merely exercise with an unnaturally longer or shorter stride you will suffer in your joints. Speed-walkers are for some reason particularly susceptible to lengthening the stride oddly. They look funny doing it and it makes hip joints, knees, and ankles hurt. Don't do it. Find your natural stride and stick with it. If you want to go faster, take more steps per minute.

If you are experiencing any strain or discomfort running bring your athletic shoes to a lesson and let your teacher watch you and help you. Better yet, bring a videotape of your exercise and watch the tape with your teacher. You will be able to analyze together what is going wrong. Keep taping and improving until you have ease and coordination.

The critical factor in running is primary control. The primary movement must be in fact primary. I mean that the movement of arms and legs in running, as in walking, must be in relation to and coordinated by the lengthening of the spine, beginning with the constant and delicate renewal of the forward and up of the head with every stride. If the spine contracts or fails to lengthen with the stride, arm and leg movement is arbitrary and unduly effortful.

If you're having trouble with walking or running review the mapping section of this book and be sure you're not mis-using your joints. Runners in trouble often find that they are dropping their pelvises down into their legs, creating an intolerable pressure in the hip joint. Others have their knees mapped too high, near the middle or top of the knee cap instead of at the bottom. Others fail to use the ankle properly. If you are hitting hard on your heel or coming down too far back on your heel, then you must rethink your whole balance. Very likely you are carrying the weight of your torso too far back in relation to your legs rather than balancing over them at the hip joint as the foot touches the ground. If you find that the rolling forward of each foot is not smooth you can be sure your torso is too far back. The foot accommodates the imbalance by staying too long at the heel. Lead with your head and shift your torso forward at the hip joints until you feel the whole back releasing as you run and the progress through the foot becoming even. When this happens you'll feel a springiness that is lovely.

Swimming

Swimmers' complaints can almost always be remedied by attention to the joint of the head and spine, the joint of the clavicle and sternum, and the joint of the leg with the pelvis. The pain and stiffness that swimmers suffer in their necks comes from tightening the neck muscles when they turn their heads to breathe, resulting in a tilting back of the head rather than a simple rotation. If the tension is severe enough that head mobility is quite limited, then it will have to be recovered by application of Alexander's principles before the swimming will improve significantly. One sign of success will be the easy resting of the head in the water when it is not being turned and the ability of the head to initiate the primary movement so that arms and legs are coordinated.

Swimmers must allow maximum movement of the clavicle and the shoulder blade in the stroke. The shoulder blade should float easily forward, as should the collarbone, making the stroke one of the entire arm structure, not just the upper arm, the lower arm, and the hand. This frees the upper back and brings the full power of the movement muscles on the back and front to the stroke.

Swimmers must kick from the joint of the thigh with the pelvis, with knees and ankles easy, not stiff. Swimmers who try to kick from the waist or there-abouts suffer lower back pain and their kicking fails to propel them through the water properly.

Bicycling

Cycling, like swimming, depends on the easy mobility of the head joint with the spine and the lengthening of the spine in response to head movement. The head must tilt back to look at traffic right at the base of the skull in such a way that the neck muscles lengthen along the cervical curve, not tighten along it, and the cyclist must maintain an easy lengthening to turn and look back. Only a lively spine will insure that the arms send weight into the handlebars without the excessive pressure that makes cyclists ache and burn across their upper backs.

Cyclists should review the part of this book that deals with the structure of the pelvis, for they must rock forward toward the handlebars with their whole torsos, not, as many do, uncomfortably, only above the waist. When move-ment forward of the whole pelvis is prevented leg power is lost. Muscles are too tied-up for power to be delivered directly into the pedal as it is if the hip joint is free.

A rather common and rather odd bit of overwork occurs when cyclists try to work on the upstroke as well as the downstroke. If the leg simply rides the upstroke and then works on the downstroke a happy cycle of rest and activity for the legs increases stamina on the long haul.

Aerobic Dance

If you want to try this, start at home. Buy a video tape of a teacher with good use and mess around with it for a few weeks on your own until you are sure that you can handle the pace and the sheer quantity of stimulus and still give yourself the attention you need to keep the movement fluid and free. If you don't feel good in a movement scrap the aerobic agenda for the moment, stop the video, rerun the movement again and again, analyze your difficulty, experiment with different ways of doing it, watch in a mirror and see what you see, in short, mess around until you get it right, then pick up the pace again and go on. Be patient with yourself. These are demanding movements. Get comfortable and safe with them before you join a class where social pressures and inadequate instruction or modeling can make the whole thing a challenge.

Or you can simplify the whole thing and just put on your favorite music and dance, gradually building to an aerobic level and adding movements of your own devising as they feel right to you. Your own moving may be less linear and more varied than the tapes. So much the better.

Exercise to Improve flexibility

If you do calisthenics or stretches or some other such system of movement to improve flexibility you have a sure measure of success or failure. Are you getting more flexible? If so, are you getting more flexible everywhere? Your spine? Your head? Your hip joint? Your ankles? Your upper arm? If so, you are no doubt doing the exercises constructively. If not, why not?

An alarming number of students come to Alexander teachers having done flexibility exercises for years without any appreciable gain. Some assume there is something wrong with them, "I'm just not flexible." Others are satisfied to keep the wolf from the door, "I'm not getting stiff like so many people my age." I suggest to my students that they needn't settle for so little. I observe that the same movements done with attention to improvement and in keeping with Alexander's discoveries can steadily increase range of motion in every joint, or at least in the joints that the exercises address. I ask students to show me their exercises every few lessons until there is sufficient improvement to liberate joints for full movement over time.

Improvement depends on adherence to simple rules. First, the student must attend to the whole body to be sure that tension somewhere other than the moving part is not limiting the movement, that, for instance, the head is not being contracted down and back when a leg is lifted. Second, the student must begin the movement with a general ease in the body. Again and again I see students do floor exercises seriously handicapped by the whole body contraction that occurred as the student dropped to the floor. I invite those students to get right back up again and repeat the moving to the floor in a manner that frees and lengthens them into the exercise position, at which time they can do the exercises with more ease and flexibility. Thirdly, the student must give the movement the support of the primary control. Spinal movements must be led by the head in a way that lengthens the spine and allows its natural sequencing to emerge, and movements of arms and legs must be reflexly supported. Faithfulness to these rules virtually guarantees increasing flexibility.

In recent years some students have expressed a longing to do flexibility work but have assumed they couldn't devote enough time to it. To one of these students I said one day, "Well, you could do worse than simply put your joints through their range of motion each day." He came back a week later and said, "I did what you suggested and it was amazing." "What was that?" I asked. "Put my joints though their range of motion each day." He showed me how much flexibility he had gained in a week doing that, and we began to systematically play with the idea. Sure enough, it works like magic and takes only about five minutes a day, with no necessity that the five minutes be consecutive. The student simply begins with the joint of the head and the spine—where else?—rotating the head and tilting, then moves on to the jaw, doing a classic whispered ah-h-h (ask your teacher about this), then on to the ribs, moving them at their joints with the vertebrae by taking a good breath. Then the student moves all four joints of the arm structure and the hand joints. Then the spine, bending forward, backward, to each side, spiraling, and twisting. Then the hip joint, knee, and ankle and the foot joints. That's it. Done correctly this routine increases flexibility faster than anything I know, and I have wondered and wondered why. I now think two factors contribute, first the quality of attention brought to the movement, which is the kind of attention that makes it possible for the body to learn from each movement. Second, some of the movements are ones that many people rarely make, like rotation at the upper arm joint with the shoulder blade and rotation at the hip joint. The body seems to delight in these movements and their availability seems to free the joint. A telling analogy: some people believe that the greatest strain on the voice is the selecting out of its full range of sound the few dozen sounds that we ordinarily make in a day. A revealing tale: some of my students have had a good range of motion in spiraling on one side and almost none on the other. How come? Once or twice a day they turned to look behind them as they backed out of their driveways.

Warm-ups

The fact is that many people are less able to move as they need to after they warm up than before. I uttered the shocking truth this baldly for the first time when I was asked in a class about warm-ups by a basketball coach. I was surprised by my bluntness, but she burst out laughing and said that day after day as she watched her team she asked herself why in the world coaches persist in warm-ups. She said she would watch young women come onto the court and start playing around with the ball, moving well and getting into it, relieved to be where they had wanted to be all day. Then she said she called the players to attention and put them through their warm-ups, after which, according to her, it took them fifteen minutes to half an hour to get back to their pre-warm-up quality of play. I subsequently taught the coach how to teach her team to put their joints through their range of motion. The team did the movements as they pleased in the first few minutes of the practice period, horsing around in the meantime as they had before. The coach told me that when practice began in earnest the team was flexible and alert. She was delighted, and she concluded that the best preparation for most activities is the gentle doing of the activity.

Stretches

Same story. Stretches done the way many people do them keep the stretchers bound up and graceless, which is a shame. If it's true of you, rethink the movements, applying the principles you have learned in this manual and from your teacher. Abandon the groaning sort of stretch for the luxurious kind that humans seem to have an inborn longing for. You'll enjoy stretching and you'll get the result you want, flexibility, suppleness.

T'ai Chi and Yoga

Lots of Alexander students and teachers are also students or teachers of t'ai chi or yoga. Two are Bruce Fertman and Martha Hanson at the Alexander Foundation in Philadelphia, who are expert in t'ai chi. Though the rest of us are willing and able to help with the direct application of Alexander's ideas to these movements, we do so as we would to any other movement, picking up a dining room chair or playing a cello, not with an eye to the development of chi or the spinal energies cultivated by yoga. The application is a valid one, I believe, because the best t'ai chi I have seen has relied as deeply on primary control as does ballet or volleyball. If you want a synthesis of the ideas, though, you must go to the experts.

Some students are puzzled by what seems to them to be a contradiction in their t'ai chi training and their Alexander training. "How can it be," they ask, "that Alexander stresses the importance of the head-spine relationship and t'ai chi the belly? Which is right?" I answer that I know a lot about primary control and next to nothing about chi, but that it does not seem strange to me that there should be more than one aspect of our being worthy of cultivation. We do not trouble ourselves that we have a circulatory system and a respiratory system in the same body with a different center of organization. We assume the two systems impinge on each other only when one is very seriously malfunctioning, and we do not go to a lung specialist when we need a cardiologist. I have no doubt that a compromised primary control interferes with the proper execution of the t'ai chi form, so I help the student restore reflex support to the movement.

Students of yoga need especially a clear understanding of the sequential nature of spinal movement, otherwise the movements fail. Take a cobra, for instance, the snake-like movement of the spine backward. If the head doesn't lead the movement, the snake-like sequencing in the movement is lost. Instead, chunks of the spinal column move at once. Those chunks get more and more frozen over time as the movement is repeated day after day, so just the opposite of the desired effect is actually achieved. Though the final posture may look convincing at first, on examination it may be seen that the student is bending mostly at the lower back. The bend is not evenly or beautifully distributed over the whole spine. Frequently the lower back is strained. I ask the student to scale the movement way back to just that movement that can truly be led by the head and to the portion of the spine that can truly sequence. This takes discipline and patience but eventually the movement can be redeemed and the spine regain its ability to sequence. The rule is: no cheating on sequence.

If You Lift Weights

If you lift weights with attention to principle you will end up with tone and strength. If you lift weights pulled down you will end up bound and stiff, and the general boundness will interfere with the application of the increased strength in particular muscles so that it will do you very little good. The difference is this: when there is ease in the whole body as the weight is lifted there can be a true isolation of the muscle group engaged. If the whole body is contracted into downward pull as the weight is lifted true isolation is impossible, so more effort lifts less weight. Alexander frees and supports the whole so that the part can function freely. Actual work increases, but effort decreases, which sometimes confuses a student. She feels half the effort and lifts twice the weight. Her question is, "Can this be doing me any good?" She has to learn that the benefit is from the work, not from the effort, and that may feel all wrong to her at first.

The biggest challenge for weight lifters in maintaining primary control is the lowering of the arms or legs, not the lifting. They seem to feel that if arms come down bodies should come down. Just the opposite is true. The easiest arm movement is supported by the gentle lengthening of the torso. If an overhead weight is being pulled down toward the body, either in front of the torso or behind it, the head should tip forward delicately so that the spine lengthens. This smoothes the movement surprisingly and removes the awkwardness.

Sports

Everything that has been said so far applies as well to a tennis serve or a golf swing or to shooting a basket. Keep the primary movement primary and you can't go wrong. Lead with your head. Maintain a unified field of attention. Think joints. Bend at your hip joints, not your waist. Allow your back to lengthen and widen in movement, transferring your weight to your spine so that your back can do the movement work it is designed to do. Protect the sequencing in your spine by freeing your neck and keeping your head poised easily on your spine. Aim for appropriate effort delivered where it counts, into the ball. Keep your body awareness bright. If you lose your fluidity get it back.

Players of sport have a resource not available to other exercisers, the models provided by television. The greatest athletes on earth can be observed and analyzed almost any hour of the day right up close where you can see exactly what they are doing. Watch your sport on TV. Watch the heads lead. Watch the spines lengthen. Watch how the fine baseball players balance over their hip joints as they pitch or bat. Stand right up in your living room and imitate it. Imitate the slight drop down and back of the head on the basketball player who missed his free-throw. Imitate the buoyant movement forward and up of the head of the next player who makes his free-throw. Imitate the kinesthetic awakeness that you see.

XIV. Sleep and Rest

Students ask again and again about sleep and rest. Some wake up stiff every morning and some wake up several times a night with pain. Some have trouble finding a comfortable position in which to fall asleep. Some are obsessed with the search for the perfect bed or the perfect pillow. Some are worried they will sleep in a wrong position. Some have been told by chiropractors that they shouldn't sleep this way or that and have trained themselves to avoid whatever it is, usually at considerable cost in effort and vigilance. Some have become reliant on various props, like bolsters under the knees or foam between the knees or sculpted head supports featuring what I secretly refer to as glacial grooves. Often the props were expensive and are inconvenient—they are extra baggage on trips—and often the relief they promised is temporary: "It helped for about a week."

Most of my students have been helped to find comfort at night and to wake up refreshed based on a few simple understandings about sleep. The first is that we are meant to move at night, like children do. Perhaps you can remember, or have current experience of, how children move at night. All over the place. Sometimes sprawled. Sometimes curled up. Sometimes with arms tucked, other times with arms akimbo. Sometimes gently shifting, sometimes flopping. Arms above the head, arms below the head, arms tucked under the body. Legs in every possible position. On the tummy. On the back. On the right side. On the left side. Everywhere in between. Head at every possible angle. Always with a quality of looseness, even when deeply, deeply asleep. Always effortlessly breathing.

We called our children flapdoodles when they crawled in with us and commandeered the whole bed by moving in the way natural to them as if there were no one else there at all. My advice is, if you have a flapdoodle in your house, learn from her how to sleep and set about reclaiming your flapdoodle nature. Encourage your sleeping partner to do the same, if you have one. Flapdoodles have a way of accommodating each other. It's the flapdoodle and the non-flapdoodle that have trouble.

Even people who used to sit for fifteen minutes on the edge of the bed working out the stiffness from the night in order to comfortably get up and make their way to a twenty minute hot shower to finish the process find they wake without stiffness or discomfort if they recover even some of their flapdoodle nature. But how is that to be done after years of rigidly adhering to two or three, or even one, positions for sleep? Well, would you believe, by attention, intention, and permission, our old friends. I recommend to people that they take some time each night before falling asleep to use what they have so far assimilated of Alexander's ideas to get as comfortable and long and easy as possible, with special attention to ease in the neck, and then to gently rehearse sleep positions. Invent them. Think of as many as you can and move into them leading with your head and letting your spine follow sequentially. This sequencing is especially important in rolling over, for it will determine whether you are free when you finish the roll, or back into an old contraction. Do not avoid the curled up positions. They are natural to us. Bodies love them, and if they are done with necks and spines long and free, they contribute to a life-long suppleness of the spine. They are your night-time yoga. As you recover your flexibility and your flapdoodleness you will find more and more positions comfortable that were before uncomfortable because of the tension in your body. So go gently through the range you find uncomfortable and visit again later.

Some of you move at night but carry through the night the tension with which you fall asleep, so your body never gets a chance to come out of its habituated contraction. You need to take a few pre-sleep moments to get your body as free as you can. Rub your neck, work along the base of your skull with your fingertips, coaxing the muscles to release. Put your hands under your skull and move your head around some, freeing it in the movement. Rest it again gently on the bed or the pillow in an easy way. Allow your whole body to fit in with that ease. Wiggle. Stretch a little in a luxurious way. Move your arms and legs, encouraging a quiet lengthening. Talk to your muscles about releasing. Then move into your favorite falling-asleep position, whatever it is, and sleep. Your body will gradually recover its customary ease in sleep.

People ask me if Alexander helps insomnia. I say maybe. Sometimes. It all depends. It all depends on the meaning and ultimate cause of the insomnia. There are people who find that increased freedom of movement and greater ease in the body are just the margin of difference, and they sleep when they would have otherwise lain awake. But there is a classic insomnia with historic or physiological causes that seems not to be alleviated by any amount of release, so there are Alexander teachers with insomnia just as there are Alexander teachers with migraines, though tension headaches have long since disappeared from their experience. Insomniacs of that sort need therapists or the attention of a sleep lab with sophisticated diagnostic equipment and treatment procedures. That is not to say that these people do not benefit from Alexander. Sometimes they say they are saved by it, for they learn that they can physically rest at a deep level even when they cannot sleep. So they lie there free and awake, which is different from tense and awake. Again, a margin of difference.

Now, on the matter of the PILLOW and the BED. What's the right bed? What's the right pillow? These questions arise again and again with astonishing urgency. One participant in a workshop told me he had spent eight thousand dollars on beds and he was contemplating yet another purchase.

What did I advise? I told him there might be some bed in heaven on which he could rest comfortably for more than a few minutes, but there is none on earth. I told him it was himself he had to change, not beds. I said the cost would be insignificant in monetary terms, but great in terms of attention to himself. I told him if he would bother to learn what we were teaching in the workshop he could eventually be comfortable on any reasonable bed. I don't know whether that particular gentleman made his way to comfort, but many have. Give up the Quest for the Bed and turn your attention to yourself. If you recover ease and movement you will be comfortable sleeping unless you have some particularly recalcitrant structural problem or injury, in which case you should work out with your teacher the accommodations necessary in your sleep to achieve the most comfort possible, some comfort being better than none.

Most Alexander students end up eventually with their pillows on the floor most mornings. Without their noticing it the pillow has ceased to be the carrier of hope. In the meantime, in the early stages of learning, the pillow may in fact be necessary. Remember that in downward pull the head is drawn forward of the spine and concurrently tilted backward. If a head in such a condition is not supported by a pillow there is a terrific strain on the area at the bottom of the cervical curve and the head rests too far up on the skull for comfort because of the chronic tilting. William Penn's mentor's advice concerning his sword was, "Carry it, lad, as long as thee can." Take a like attitude toward your pillow. Use it as long as thee need it or want it.

The cervical pillow is tricky. It provides essential support during healing from some injuries, like whiplash. But it is another piece of paraphernalia that can be misused and thereby increase discomfort. One kind of damaging misuse of it is contracting across it, in which case the head is drawn down and back over it and downward pull is exaggerated. If you use a cervical pillow you must free your neck muscles and lengthen gently along its curve. In some people this actually serves as a useful mapping tool. These people are never tempted to think they should have a straight neck, and they learn what it is to lengthen along a curve in the body, which ultimately helps them get the hang of lengthening along the thoracic curve and the lumbar curve as well. The other misuse is staying glued to it and failing to move into other positions, which slows healing and promotes stiffness. People who need the pillow for a time get used to reaching for it whenever they return to their backs in sleep from other positions, which is, of course, when they need it.

Some students confess in hushed tones that they read in bed, expecting I guess to be told they must never do it again and if they do their fingers will fall off. Instead, if they are in fact uncomfortable reading in bed we retrain the reclining so that they are supported and long and so that they have several different positions to roam among as they read.

Rest

I'm convinced that left to our own devices we would continue to intersperse bursts of activity with little rests as we did as children and as animals do. Alexander teachers rely on little periods of "lying-down work" during the day which are wondrously refreshing. Recipes for this "work" vary like recipes for chocolate cake. They're all good. The common ingredients are lying on the back, lengthening and widening and releasing like mad, with the knees up. The head is supported by a book, if you like. I love to roll my head around on a four inch rubber ball right at the base of my skull. This would be regarded as pretty peculiar by many of my colleagues, but they haven't tasted my chocolate cake with scotch and raisins, either. One keeps "directing," as the English Alexander teachers call it, which means intending a release of one's head out of its contraction down and back and a consequent releasing throughout the spine and the arm structure and the legs, plus a thousand other releases as you wish. There will be a quality of letting go, but with a difference. Letting go can remain pretty local and can become hydra-headed. Releasing, by contrast, has a unifying effect, for one is releasing into a profound level of psychophysical organization.

Within the period of rest many of us do "whispered ah-h-h-hs," a simple, restful, effective means of releasing the breathing and the jaw and the throat which was devised by Alexander himself. Various detailed descriptions of this procedure are in the literature elsewhere. In any case, it is best to learn it from one's teacher. Just ask.

If you don't have five minutes to devote to constructive rest, as the lying-down-work I've just described is sometimes called, you can return to rest in activity at any time. Just come home to your kinesthesia, release into your primary control as into a pair of slippers, take a good wide breath, and carry on.

A word of caution. Don't abuse these rest techniques by using them to allay the effects of chronic overwork, which they will do, up to a point. Small alternations of rest and activity do not substitute for larger ones, which we also need.

XV. The Technique and Common Maladies

I often imagine conversations with F. M. Alexander. One fantasy involves his calling me on the telephone. He tells me that he's an actor and he has had the problem that he has repeatedly lost his voice. He says someone told him that I might be able to help him. "Do you think you could help me?" he asks. I tell him that I have certainly helped others in his situation, and I hope I will be able to help him. I ask him whether his problem has been medically evaluated. I hear rather an earful in answer to that question. He's not diseased, he says. I say in that case we may make an appointment, and we do. I often imagine his lessons, his quickness, his eagerness, his rather overwhelming personality, his perseverance, his delight, his reciting his beloved Shakespeare in his later lessons.

Future generations of teachers will teach those who learn for pleasure, prevention, and peak performance. The current generation teaches mostly people like F. M., impaired but not diseased, those who suffer from the maladies of misuse, such as back pain, carpal tunnel syndrome, tension headaches, vocal problems, temporomandibular joint (TMJ) problems, fibromyalgia, (the relatively new diagnosis, the ubiquitous one; not the old diagnosis of the fairly rare condition that makes palpable little knots in the muscles; the new diagnosis appears to be Latin for *tense*) and thoracic outlet syndrome. These problems tend to disappear when primary control is recovered and the student's body is correctly mapped.

What should a person do who is suffering from a use-induced malady? Change. That's what F. M. Alexander did, and he got his voice back full-force and secure. He observed his misuse; he analyzed his misuse so that he understood the nature of the change he must make; he inhibited his habitual misuse; he cooperated with the emerging improved use; and then he celebrated. He learned it was the misuse of the whole of him that was affecting the part of him, that is, his downward pull affected his voice. (If he had been a secretary he might have turned up with carpal tunnel; if he played the flute, TMJ; if he made stained glass, thoracic outlet syndrome; etc.) As the whole improved, the part improved. With good use, the parts tend to lose vulnerability.

Alexander teachers can often significantly help people with injuries, but that's another matter altogether. Whiplash is a good example. The Technique helps release the spasm that occurred on impact. It is normal for muscle to spasm to stabilize an injured joint, but in whiplash, spasm tends to continue long after its usefulness and itself becomes a problem which lessons can gently relieve.

XVI. Stage-Fright and the Alexander Technique

People often ask about the application of Alexander's ideas to what is fashionably called performance anxiety. My one answer: embody the fear. Persons are only overwhelmed by fear in a way that impairs performance when the fear is not grounded or when a person is not willing to feel the fear in its totality. Any attempt not to feel the fear splits the performer psychically into two persons, the feeler and the repressor. It is the splitting, not the fear, that limits capability. Worse, performers will reduce their body awareness in an attempt to reduce their fear. They want to avoid the intense sensation of their fear, so they numb out. It is the numbing and not the fear that limits capacity. It is the attempt not to feel rather than the feeling that impairs performance.

The autobiographies of many great performers describe in vivid detail the agonies of fear their authors experienced before they walked on stage. The performers stood there and felt their fear, and when they walked on stage embodied and awake the fear was gradually transformed into the energy for performance.

Frank Jones used to say that anything can be regarded as the stimulus to which you choose the response of lengthening and freeing. That's what I've seen Michael Jordan do in relation to the last five seconds of a tied game with seventeen million people watching him. It's what an actor or a singer may do in response to a wave of fear. Just go up in response to it.

When a person actually apprehends and acknowledges that freeing and lengthening is a possible response to a wave of fear (something we may readily observe in wildlife) then that person is in a position in retrospect to understand that pulling down was a response to fear, not an expression of it. Expressions of fear are: trembling, watchfulness, emitting fearful sounds, readiness to flee or fight, and the like. Pulling down is not an expression of fear but rather a resistance to it. Pulling down dulls sensation, including the sensation of emotion. A surprising number of students have learned this fact prior to their Alexander Technique lessons and a surprising number of students use it consciously, as, "I scrunch my body in order not to feel," or, "I tighten up when I get scared and then I don't feel so scared." I recommend that students keep this behavior in their repertoire. Circumstances may arise in which the behavior is life-preserving; but performance anxiety is not such a circumstance. Performance anxiety has to be felt full-out and responded to constructively or performance suffers.

There's another, related matter. Sometimes it turns out that it is not fear at all that a performer is dealing with, but rather inner talk, a litany of self-deprecating voices. These, too, can be embodied and treated as a stimulus for freeing, but this is a more serious condition, because it is rare for the energy of those voices to be transmuted into the energy of performance, as fear is. The tendency toward self-deprecation has antecedents in the past, whereas the fear is of the moment. For this condition therapy may be necessary to resolve the pressure of the past on the present.

XVII. If You Have Suffered Abuse or Violence

If you were a victim of child abuse or other violence you will find the Alexander Technique a crucial aid in recovery. Survivors must win back their birthright—emotion, memory, self-knowledge, self-love, embodiment. The body is both the goal and the means in this victory, and the technique is a means to the means.

Teachers who work with victims in their recovery gain a profound respect for the healing process as it emerges in each person uniquely, in a way quite specifically suited to the nature and degree of the hurt and to the innate qualities of the person healing. The Alexander Technique's contribution to a healing process is, first, increased awareness, which is of supreme importance in healing because victims of violence without exception numb themselves in order to function. Since the Alexander Technique is something you learn rather than something that is done to you, you can pace your increasing awareness. If you have been fearful of being overwhelmed by the sensation of repressed emotion in your body you can develop kinesthesia so that as emotion emerges it is grounded in the senses and finds expression in them that is safe.

The Alexander Technique offers you constructive conscious control. This is an aspect of the work that survivors often prize even more than other persons because it gives choice where before there was no choice. The aspect of constructive conscious control called inhibition is particularly useful to people who are healing from hurt. Those who, as a result of the harm done to them, often at an early age, are susceptible to addiction or to abuse of themselves or self destruction, or who fear that they may be harmful to others as a result of projected rage, are grateful to learn that they can stop and reconsider. Increased body awareness leads to increased self awareness and self awareness leads naturally to an altered sense of time in which there are opportunities for pausing. When we pause we may reconsider and say no to what we were about to do, or we can wait. Persons learn that waiting is the condition in which something constructive is likely to emerge, naturally, out of the vast inventive potential that always waits underneath harm to re-emerge, like a tulip in spring. Persons who are healing learn to become very skillful inhibitors, not in the sense that they do nothing, but in the sense that they say no to habituated self destruction and wait for the more constructive response that was blocked by the habitual.

The Alexander Technique offers you an opportunity to build a new trust in yourself and your body. As you explore the body's wonderful architecture you come to know that the body is meant to feel not numb and not miserable but good. At the same time, as you allow your body to express despair or fear or rage you gain a regard for the body's expressive powers and its ability to free itself. That trust engenders self-care. Self-care is a challenge survivors must learn to meet. Their tendency is to perpetuate the care they were given, not the care they require. Trust and appreciation lead naturally to self-care, breaking the cycle of neglect, deprivation, and heartache.

XVIII. The Relationship of the Alexander Technique to Somatic Techniques

Over the last few decades a new field of inquiry has arisen called somatics. The field's development has taken a course opposite to many fields. Rather than branching into specializations from a common core of information as medicine and chemistry did, somatics began specialized and has gradually generalized as workers in one discipline have become curious about other disciplines. Most persons in the field look for an integration of somatic disciplines over the next few generations.

One might make an analogy to a jigsaw puzzle. Here and there unrelated persons discovered pieces of the body puzzle. Gradually the pieces have come together and are fitting together. Alexander discovered a corner piece of the body puzzle, one of the really important pieces that orients the others.

There is another model of somatics that is instructive. In her book *Somatics: Perspectives on the Emerging Field of Psychophysical Integration*, Wendy Morris draws a continuum with Somatic Therapy on one end and Somatic Education on the other. The Alexander Technique leads the column at the Education end of the continuum, Structural-Functional Educators. Body-oriented psychotherapists are at the Therapy end of the continuum, with dance therapists, energetic therapists, and body awareness educators in between. (Wendy Morris's excellent book can be ordered from her at 2416 34th Avenue South, #2, Minneapolis MN 55406.) Her model emphasizes the Technique as education, or, as many of us prefer, re-education.

I believe that it is accurate to say that most Alexander Technique teachers regard the Technique as one bright strand in the large braid of somatics, but some do not. Some want to claim a status for the Technique as unique, outside somatics, and rightly understood only in contrast to other disciplines. In this argument the teachers look not to the results (they acknowledge that many techniques result in greater freedom and ease of movement and the recovery of body awareness) but to the means. No other method features constructive conscious control, the cognitive process that Alexander used to recover his freedom.

Constructive conscious control exploits the brain's vast potential for consciousness of self and for choice. Some prominent neuroscientists believe that self-consciousness (in the good sense) and choice depend on the size and structure of the human brain. Both the size and the structure make it possible for the brain to process its own functioning (creatures with smaller, differently structured brains cannot do this), resulting in consciousness. Alexander's Technique uses the brain consciously for self-observation of habitual use of the organism, for conscious inhibition of habitual use, for conscious observation of an emerging more integrated use, for conscious cooperation with the more integrated use, and even for conscious observation of the more integrated use, all this depending surely on the conscious linking of conceptual and motor functions in the brain, by choice. Rather than creating a split, as some might expect, all this consciousness instead has a profoundly integrating effect, healing the split many people experience between thinking and being, or mind and body, or consciousness and functioning. It is this integration which is the great good the Technique offers, with freedom and ease as by-products, according to the argument we are exploring.

History will resolve this debate. Here's my view. The Alexander Technique should disappear eventually, not into somatics, but into education. The Alexander Technique, including all that has been learned about primary control and constructive conscious control, should be integrated as the alphabet and numbers have been. Someone(s) discovered/invented the alphabet and numbers once, which now are in general use. May it someday be the same for primary control and constructive conscious control.

XIX. How to Choose your Alexander Teachers

Alexander teachers vary in competence in the same proportion as other professionals, it seems to me. You will, of course, want to seek out excellent teachers, who will usually come highly recommended by someone you trust. If you don't know anyone who knows the teacher(s) in your area, just go have a first lesson and keep careful track of your experience. If you leave the lesson lighter and easier, more mobile, more sensitive kinesthetically, breathing easier, more aware of your surroundings, with a greater sense that you have choice about your physical responses to stimuli, then you have found a good teacher and you can safely consider taking a series of lessons.

You will be able to tell a great deal, though not everything, by how your teacher moves. Look for ease and alertness and balance. The fact is that most Alexander teachers came to the Technique to solve problems of their own. In the course of working on themselves many persons become so interested in the body and in the function of constructive conscious control in relation to it that they decide to become teachers. Those persons become good teachers and their experience of liberating themselves is an asset to their students. The teachers have a real understanding of what the student is going through. The student is better off because the teacher has solved her own problems. The late Judy Leibowitz is a well-known example of such a teacher. Leibowitz dramatically improved the movement in her own body which had been handicapped by polio and went on to become a powerful and empathetic teacher. If you ask your teacher about her own experience of the Technique you may hear a heroic story. Remember that the teacher is teaching the process of physical liberation and the recovery of primary control and constructive conscious control. In this work the very process that takes one from A to B takes one from M to N and from Y to Z. The degree of freedom at any given moment is not the point so much as clarity about the process. The relevant question is: can this teacher teach me the process by which I free myself?

Something must be said about the means that the teacher uses in the teaching. There are a set of what have become known as traditional procedures in Alexander teaching. One is table work, or tablework. Chair work, or chairwork. There is the monkey, and the lunge, and hands-on-the-back-of-the-chair and there is the whispered a-h-h. Some teachers use all of these procedures and some use a few of them sometimes and some use none of them. The quality of your teacher does not depend in any way on the use of the traditional procedures. There are excellent teachers who use them and excellent teachers who do not. There is tremendous variation in what the teachers actually do in the traditional work. I have, in fact, never seen any two teachers work in exactly the same way, though training schools tend to produce teachers who are more similar to each other than they are to graduates of other schools. There are definite styles among teachers.

Chair work and table work take their character from the object supporting the student. In the table work the student lies on a table not unlike a massage table, sometimes padded, sometimes not, depending on the teacher, usually but not always with a book or several books under the student's head. The teacher works with the student's head, freeing the student's neck, bringing the student's head to a more felicitous relationship with the spine. The changed relationship will always start a process of freeing and lengthening down the spine, a widening and lengthening of the whole back, and a release of the limbs, which the teacher then carries on to fuller experience, often though not always working directly with the limbs and lower back. Usually the student remains in a supine position, that is, on her back, but many teachers now work also with the prone position and some positions in between prone and supine. The student is variously instructed. Some teachers ask their students to simply go on inhibiting their old responses while the teacher initiates a new experience in the student's body. Some teachers want their students to go on repeating Alexander's orders for the neck to free so that the head may move forward and up so that the back may lengthen and widen. Some teachers want the student to give the teacher the weight of the limbs as the limbs are moved and other teachers want the students to be doing the moving but doing it in a new way which the student discerns from the guidance of the teacher's hands.

Some teachers talk very little during work with traditional procedures and some talk a lot. Verbal processing of kinesthetic experience is wonderfully helpful to the student, but it is not the only good way to teach. Some Alexander teachers are not particularly verbal people. They invite processing with their hands, or they rely on the body to assimilate something even if it is not named. If you are getting freer and more awake and more able to choose free movement you are being taught well. It might be interesting to you, and useful, to talk to your teacher about her teaching style, about why she makes the choices she makes.

Chair work varies from style to style. In some cases the teacher will stand behind the student and guide the freeing movement of the head and the lengthening of the spine. Often the teacher sits in a chair next to the student in order to work with the arms or in front of the student to help thighs and knees and ankles fit in with the lengthening. In other cases there is a very active moving of the student in and out of the chair and a very active directing up that nevertheless for the student has a profoundly involuntary quality that some people love and some people hate and some people value sometimes as an adjunct to subtler work. You can decide for yourself if you study with a teacher who works in that way. Again, the style is not the question. All styles done well promote freedom. The only question is, are you getting freer?

Monkey and lunge and hands-on-the-back-of-the-chair are positions of mechanical advantage that can be used to learn about all similar movements in life. Monkey is any of the positions a human assumes anywhere between being fully upright and being in a deep squat. The monkey closest to upright is referred to as a shallow monkey, and the monkey closest to a full squat is called a deep monkey. The torso is bent forward at the hip joint at an angle always proportional to the bending of the knees. The body is balanced over the arch of the foot and the knees are tending slightly out over the toes. You may remember that little children spend huge amounts of time in monkeys of various depths and use squatting for many of their purposes close to the ground. Nothing can be more useful to a student than regaining the ability to squat. It liberates everything. F. M. Alexander is in a shallow monkey in the picture near the beginning of the manual. Many Alexander teachers encourage students to begin many activities by coming "up from monkey," meaning going into monkey and then coming to upright, looking for balance. The uprightness the student achieves carries the advantages of the squat, lively legs and a lively back.

The lunge is a sideways monkey with the weight on one leg, simply how humans move until they are taught not to. The lunge is the lunge cultivated in tennis as the player comes out of the monkey in which she waits for the serve, and in the martial arts, taking advantage of the power of the legs and the springiness of the torso in forward movements or in turning movements at that angle.

Hands-on-the-back-of-the-chair is just what it sounds like. I have seen many variations on the theme. Some are done sitting and some in monkey. Some teachers advocate one position of the wrist and fingers and some teachers another, but in any case the position provides unending opportunity to lengthen the arms, free across the upper back, extend the fingers without effort, widen the back of the hands, learn to make real contact without tightening, learn about the rotation of the lower arm, feel the continuity from the tip of the little finger on back through the arm to the tip of the shoulder blade, and much more.

The whispered ah-h-h is an activity carried out to free the throat and jaw and tongue and coordinate the primary control with exhalation. It's a marvelous thing. There are as many whispered ah-h-hs as there are Alexander teachers, nearly as many as there are varieties of apples in New York State. They all work, because teachers tend to come up with a personal variety that is truly useful to their students or they abandon it altogether because it requires great patience to teach it well. If your teacher teaches it, it will be good for you.

Many teachers teach the lunge and monkey constantly without ever appearing to. If a teacher helps you pick up your baby's toys off the floor in a mechanically advantageous way, bending at your ankles, knees, and hip joints and initiating your primary control going down and going up, your teacher is teaching you monkey. The basic principles are all there. If your teacher helps you with your t'ai chi you will do many lunges and monkeys right in the course of the form. Teachers who use the Dart procedures foster all the virtues of monkey and lunge. Indeed, monkey is built into almost all the Dart movements in some way.

Similarly it is possible to teach everything about the hands and arms that hands-on-the-back-of-the-chair teaches with the hand on a violin bow. And many teachers promote all the freeing of the whispered ah-h-h with other vocal material, such as the singing of Happy Birthday. Do you see that it is not the form but the content that matters? Not the form but the freeing.

In my opinion the biggest difference in teachers is their willingness or unwillingness to work directly in the activity that is important in your life. Some teachers love to work with musicians at their instruments, applying Alexander's discoveries directly to the requirements of the instrument. Others insist that the student make the application himself from his work in the chair or in monkey. Both methods work to free a musician. I am a strong advocate of what has come to be called working in activity. If you are having trouble freeing your neck when you ride your bicycle then I invite you to bring your bicycle right into the teaching room or we go into the street and I watch you ride and coach the needed changes. I go to students' spas with them and to their pottery wheels. I get a kick out of direct application, and progress is rapid, but it is not the only way. Many students have transferred what they learned in whispered ah-h-hs with their teachers to every element of their singing and done very well. The only criterion is freedom.

If you are a performing artist looking for help from the Alexander Technique, you may want to find a teacher who performs. There are splendid active artists among Alexander Technique teachers. You can learn a great deal by attending their performances and by asking them to demonstrate in your lessons. In addition, there are teachers who are experienced in teaching performers though they themselves do not perform. I keep a list of teachers experienced in teaching musicians which you can procure by sending me a stamped self-addressed envelope. The teachers on the list are self-selected and describe their work in their own words.

You will want to know whether and how your teacher uses bodies of information outside the Technique. There are teachers who are also Physical Therapists. They have a great advantage in teaching injured people because of their P. T. training. They are free to prescribe equipment and procedures that may speed healing. There are also Alexander Technique teachers who are Feldenkrais practitioners. Others are Laban trained. This is added richness. All good teachers readily identify what comes from other sources in their teaching and how it relates to the Technique.

People ask about certification of teachers. You will read that you should study only with a certified teacher. The fact is there are wonderful teachers who are certified and there are wonderful teachers who are not because the politics of certification is as strange in the Alexander world as politics often is.

There is a better criterion than certification, and that is training. You certainly want a trained teacher. Competent Alexander teaching takes a long arduous training or a very special very rare talent. F. M. Alexander taught his brother A. R. Alexander to be a fine teacher very quickly, according to legend, but A. R. had no doubt been thinking about and observing the things his brother was learning for a very long time. The thinking must have been profound and the observation acute. The legend should not be used to justify inadequate training.

There are approved trainings and non-approved trainings in almost every country that has Alexander teachers. The approval comes from the professional organization that has achieved ascendancy in the country or claimed it by default. In those organizations there is legitimate concern for quality and a continuing attempt to assure quality of teaching. The guidelines set for training are sound ones and should be honored. Nonetheless, some non-approved courses continue to turn out competent teachers with extensive, high-quality training. Reality is always messy. To complicate things further, there are teachers who believe that Alexander teachers should be licensed as massage therapists now are, and there are Alexander teachers who think licensing is the worst thing that could happen to the profession. The latter believe that licensing insures a relentless decline in quality. The matters of certification and licensing will come to some resolution, good or bad, in some future time.

In the meantime, what to do? Stick to principle. The Alexander promise is psychophysical integrity. Any competent teacher will help you along that path.

In the United States there are two professional organizations for Alexander teachers, the North American Society for the Teachers of the Alexander Technique, or N.A.S.T.A.T., and Alexander Technique International, or A.T.I.

The former is comprised of teachers who came from N.A.S.T.A.T. approved trainings or those who joined by a process of peer review. A.T.I. is made up mostly but not entirely of persons from non-affiliated trainings, which is a term more descriptive of the reality than non-approved trainings, for certainly the A.T.I. trainings are self-approved and peer-approved. The quality distribution is about the same in both N.A.S.T.A.T. and A.T.I. as far as I can see. If your teacher belongs to either organization you have a shot at quality. And there are excellent teachers who belong to neither.

To request teacher lists for the United States write or call:

N.A.S.T.A.T.	A.T.I.
P.O. Box 517	1692 Massachusetts Ave.
Urbana, IL 61801	Cambridge, MA 02138
tel. 800-473-0620	tel. 617-497-2242
http://www.alexandertech.org	http://www.ATI-net.com

Both of these Web pages are good places to start exploring for Alexander-related materials. Each includes teacher listings, references to books and articles, and links to many other sites.

Appendix I. Origins and Theory of Mapping

This chapter is revised from a paper presented by William Conable at the Third International Alexander Congress in Engelberg, Switzerland in August, 1991. It is printed in its original form in the Congress papers, published by Direction, Bondi, Australia, 1992.

Introduction

Our ideas about body mapping are not central to understanding the Technique, nor do they substitute for its essential teachings: primary control, inhibition, orders, and the like; but they can be important pedagogical tools. They are also not wholly original with us. They are clearly implied in Alexander's writings; both of our principal teachers, Marjorie Barstow and Frank Pierce Jones, occasionally used them in teaching us. They are suggested in David Gorman's work and in the pedagogy of many of our colleagues. What this chapter hopes to contribute is systematic exploration and a theoretical framework.

In trying to understand the difficulties people have in learning the Alexander Technique it is useful to observe that the words by which we refer to the parts of our bodies do not mean the same thing to all of us. This being true, what we do to carry out intentions related to the parts of our bodies is not consistent among all of us. This can easily be demonstrated in any group of people by asking them to point to their *shoulders* or their *hips*. Even among people very sophisticated in their appreciation of the human body (such as Alexander teachers) there is often a wide range of answers to such a question. It is noteworthy that in general all of these answers will be correct—that is, they will each refer to what people sometimes agree that these words mean.

Alexander frequently referred to what he called people's "imperfect sensory appreciation." What did he mean by this term? Although sometimes he maintains that he is referring to all the senses, the main thrust of his discussion refers to kinesthesis. There are two possible sources of the distortion Alexander describes. The first is that undue pressure on or tension in the kinesthetic receptors leads to a distortion of the information they send back to the brain; or perhaps that by the phenomenon of sensory accommodation the information they send is screened out. This is, in other words, the transmission of an imperfect or "debauched" kinesthetic message to the centers where it is interpreted.

The second possibility is that the information sent to the brain is indeed accurate, but is misinterpreted in experience. This would lay the emphasis in

Alexander's statement on the word *appreciation*. This second possibility is the subject of this chapter.

Body Maps

We all seem to have in our minds *maps* of our bodies and their workings. They include size, shape, and mechanics. These maps are what we use to interpret our kinesthetic and visceral sensations; at least to some extent, we also guide our movement by them. This is not the same thing as the well-known neurological correspondence of various parts of the brain to various parts of the body. That is simply physiological; the map being discussed here is something constructed in consciousness.

The function of creating these maps may be in some way innate, but their contents are not. It is easy to understand that this must be so. Our bodies change in size and shape so radically and so continually throughout the course of our lives that if our maps of them could not change, the maps would almost always be erroneous.

Because the maps must be able to be changed, they must be learned. They are created from the experience of movement, of touching and being touched, and maybe from other things as well. They are our memories of our *interpretations* of our experience. But because these interpretations may not be accurate, the maps based on them may also not be accurate.

Indeed, inaccuracy in this regard seems almost inevitable. Knowledge of the complex details of the structure and function of the human body is not available to an infant mapping his or her body. Misunderstood or erroneous verbal and pictorial information, imitation of others' idiosyncrasies, and emotional charging or rejection of various body parts may play a distorting role. Fantasy and simple guessing are important sources for the details of the map. Details may be mistaken; neither is there any guarantee that the map will be consistent. Since it is formed out of many experiences over a long period of time and on the basis of an incomplete awareness of the totality of the body (or indeed, of the self) it is quite usual for different aspects of the body map to be, if not grossly contradictory, at least subtly inconsistent.

It also seems to be true that the interpretations forming the basis of the map are often unconsciously performed. They often take place early in life, well before the development of a sophisticated adult consciousness. Therefore the map based on them is often at least partly unconscious and often initially accessible to adult scrutiny only with some difficulty. Once this difficulty is overcome, it is possible to learn to change the map with surprising ease and with surprisingly powerful results.

An Example

The following story is a good introduction to the use of the mapping concept (in fact the incident led me to develop the idea) and illustrates a number of its implications. Some years ago a colleague asked me to observe a violin student who was having difficulty bending her bow arm at the elbow. Nothing the student or the teacher could think of was effective in helping her to solve this problem. Watching her play, I asked myself what I would have to think in order to move that way. It looked to me as if a possible answer was that she was thinking of her elbow joint about two inches higher on her arm than it really was. I thought that a plausible reason for this would be that that was the distance of her elbow from her shoulder when she started the violin as a child and that perhaps she had not changed her thinking as she grew.* When I proposed this to her and showed her where her elbow joint really moved, she said, "Oh, I can do that," and immediately proceeded to play with a freely moving elbow.

This story is significant in several ways. first is the issue of how the student's map influenced her behavior. Because she felt her elbow joint to be located where in truth there was nothing but solid bone, when she tried to bend it there no movement could occur. Further, since she interpreted the sensations from the area where the joint actually existed as being in the middle of her forearm, it became important for her to prevent any movement *there*—if you bend in the middle of a bone, something is broken! *Yet the moment she was made aware of these unconscious assumptions and revised them, she was able to move in a very different way.* This reveals an important underlying principle which seems to operate consistently: if there is a conflict between the way the body is mapped and the way it actually is, people will behave as if the map were true. I believe that this is because the map is the interface between conscious awareness and the bodily mechanisms: it is literally how we know ourselves. Although it is amenable to observation on a meta-level of consciousness, most of the time we simply accept it. And yet such is the power of the mapping function that simply changing the map can effect an instantaneous change in experience and behavior.

Next it is interesting that although this student was apparently unable to bend her elbow when playing the violin, she bent it over and over again in other activities of her life: eating, combing her hair, driving a car, and so on. This illustrates the apparent fact that the body map need not be internally consistent. In this it is no different from any other mental representation that people make of the world. Indeed, by its very nature any mental representation of the world is not the same as what it represents, and thus is necessarily flawed. Much of the time this is insignificant and even beneficial; sometimes it leads to difficulties.

---

* I am no longer confident of this interpretation. I now believe it more likely that the student was interpreting the kinesthetic sensations from the triceps tendon as if they came from the elbow joint itself; but the results were the same, both for the student and for my future thinking.

Types of Mismapping

There are various common types of mapping errors. People map their bodies erroneously as regards size, structure, and function; they leave things out; and they are prone to vagueness and blankness. Illustrating these sorts of problems allows the discussion of a number of interesting examples without the necessity of offering a detailed description of the complete map.

Size is one of the most widespread inaccuracies in the map. A particularly prevalent mismapping is a result of the adolescent growth spurt. At the very time when rapid changes are occurring in the size, shape, and proportions of the body (and thus when the map is in strong need of revision) typical American students spend hours sitting still in school. The map is unconsciously revised through experience of movement and contact: the two things least likely to happen in junior high school. If this were not enough, children of this age are likely to feel awkward or self-conscious about their bodies and bewildered by their changing sexuality, as it affects both their internal and their social experience. Small wonder that many of us responded by saying in effect "Body? What body? I don't want to know about it!" and thus interfered with the automatic re-mapping process at a crucial developmental moment.

This can be observed in the demeanor of gawky adolescents of both sexes, awkwardly trying to operate an adult-sized body on the basis of a child-sized map. Sometimes they try to force the body down to the size their self-concept tells them it is—we often try to adjust the territory to fit the map!—stooping to get the head down to the level of smaller peers, or pulling the shoulders down in a way that gives the impression of a huge long neck on a spindly body. The hip joints are often operated as if they were the old distance from the head, and there seems to be no right place for the arms. Strange distortions are imposed in an effort to increase or decrease the size of the body as a whole or of various parts which are considered too large or too small. Many of these awkwardnesses are gradually eliminated as the map is unconsciously revised; but many adults manifest the discomforts of early adolescence in their body maps through life.

Other examples of sizing errors have other sources. We have found that most people greatly underestimate the diameter of the spine. When asked to demonstrate the size of one of their own cervical vertebrae, people will typically show diameters ranging from two to four centimeters. Rarely will anyone get close to the true dimension (a minimum of five cm. for a small adult) and almost everyone is astonished when shown how to feel the transverse processes of his or her own atlas. Realizing the true size of the spinal column gives almost anyone an increased sense of strength and stability.

The most frequent example of structural mismapping is the wrong location of joints. The story of the violin student above is an instance of this problem.

Another common example which effects musicians and others who depend on finger dexterity is the mislocation of the joint between the proximal phalanges of the fingers and their respective metacarpals. This is not placed at the line at the base of the fingers (on the palm side) but from one to two centimeters further down into the palm. Going back in forth in one's mind between these two maps and wiggling the fingers is a highly revealing experiment in the power of the map.

The words *hip* and *shoulder* each have several meanings in English, and it is quite common for people to think of the hip and shoulder *joints* in ways which combine several of these meanings. People often try to move their arms as if there were no sterno-clavicular or gleno-humeral joints but at a notional joint at the inner border of the deltoid muscle (see the drawing on page 53). Similarly, they try to move their legs from the very top of the pelvis, or from an imagined joint at the bottom of the ischia or at the pelvic attachment of the gracilis muscle. Each of these misconceptions has its own characteristically distorted gait. There are dozens more of these confusions about joint placement.

Functional misconceptions also abound. One very common one is important for people who practice manual skills. When the forearm is rotated, the ulna is stable, while the radius rotates around it. This creates an axis of rotation approximately in line with the little finger. Few people realize this, but instead try to stabilize the radius and rotate the ulna on a putative axis in line with the thumb, the first finger, or the middle finger. This mistake can cause severe problems of awkwardness and even tendinitis.

The last kind of mapping errors which I will mention are those of vagueness, blankness, or absence of a part of the body in the map. These lacunae can come from simple ignorance or imitation. Frequently, however, they are the result of withdrawing from an injury and never entirely re-establishing contact with the injured part. Also, unfortunately, they can be the result of physical or psychological abuse which leads the sufferer to disown or distort part of the body. In such cases there may be a resistance to correcting the map, or there may be a resurfacing of repressed traumatic experiences which requires emotional support or treatment as an adjunct to the work of the teacher.

Appendix II. If You're an Instrumentalist

The best kept secret among instrumentalists is that they move for a living. Not only do they move for a living, they do the most complex moving done by humans. Yet few of the insights into movement and how to improve movement that have come out of somatics in the past few decades have made their way into the training of musicians. Most music teaching is still done without attention to the movement aspects of making music.

The result of this lack is that many musicians are in trouble—they are in pain as they play or they suffer technical limitation. The most visible resource available to them in their difficulties is the music medicine community. These physicians and physical therapists are exactly what is needed for the small percentage of musicians who genuinely have a medical problem but they are usually inadequate for that majority of cases where the issue is misuse.

The body is beautifully designed for repetitive movement unless it is misused. Statistics confirm this, for though forty percent of musicians experience pain in playing, sixty percent do not. If repetitive movement were the issue, all musicians should hurt. Our observation is that musicians who hurt misuse themselves. They exhibit classic downward pull or they have faulty maps or they have limited kinesthesia and do not notice that they are using more effort than they need or they misunderstand how something is done.

When neck muscles tighten there are consequences in two directions, up and down. You already know the worst consequence above the neck, the displacement of the head off its poise on the spine and the resulting tension and restricted mobility. The musicians who suffer most directly from the loss of mobility of the head are violinists and flute players. A violinist's plight is addressed here as an example of the appropriateness of movement analysis.

There are four sources of support for the violin: the violin-shelf (the collarbone), the left arm and hand, the stabilizing trajectory of the bow, and the weight of the head. Repeat: the weight of the head, by which is meant *only* the weight of the head. Too many violinists are in trouble because they don't understand this. They believe they must *work* with their heads in relation to the violin, so they tighten their necks. Think about it. A head weighs eight to fifteen pounds and a violin less than two. The weight alone is sufficient to prevent the violin's falling to the floor, especially since the other sources of support are available much of the time. The stability of the collarbone is always available. A violinist must keep the neck muscles free so that the weight of the head may effortlessly release onto the violin when the weight is needed. Repeat: *when the weight is needed*. Often the finest players take the weight of the head off the violin when the weight isn't needed, which is much of the time. When the weight is required it should be in proportion as the other sources of support are not available. If a violinist is starting way up the fingerboard and must shift down into a lower position, then the weight of the head must be dropped onto the chinrest to stabilize the violin. But later when the gesture is over and the music has changed, then the head may come off the violin. There should be a constant interplay of the four sources of support—collarbone, arm, head, and bow—depending entirely on the requirements of the music. What the music will never require is tension in the muscles of the neck.

Violinists in trouble often have powerful habits that prevent the easy release of weight onto the violin. They must work consciously on bringing the violin into playing position by inhibiting their old habits so that something more constructive can happen. They begin by finding all the awareness and ease available to them at the moment. Then they bring the violin up to the violin-shelf using the movement to enhance awareness and to enhance primary control by gently lengthening. That gentle lengthening as the violin comes up seems to be instinctive in the great violinists, and it can be learned. I ask violinists to bring the violin up without moving the head toward it and without raising the bow arm. They sometimes take ten or fifteen tries before the tendency to automatically go lurching toward the violin with the head can be inhibited. The players will laugh at the power of their habits, at how silly it seems that they can't just not do that lurching. Once they have brought their violins up without engaging the old head habits they need to repeat this new use until the arm movement and the head movement are no longer so associated.

If the player releases the head delicately forward and up as she brings her head to the violin she will get a gentle lengthening of the spine at the same time. She then gets not only stability for the violin but also the whole-body support of the primary control for arm and body movement. Then magic is possible, for that is what the greats do—they release the weight of their heads onto the violin in such a way that the spinal reflexes that support their playing are stimulated. Two for the price of one.

I focused first on the violin because of the role of the head in violin playing, though I hope you understand that a free neck and a balanced head are essential for every instrument. The point I have wanted to make is this: we always keep the primary control primary. Then, as we keep the primary control primary we give attention to mechanical integrity in all the parts and retrain the part within the whole whenever and wherever that is necessary so that a musician can play easily and comfortably.

My intention eventually is to write a detailed description of the application of the Technique and of body mapping to each orchestral instrument and some others. All I can do here is give you a whiff of what's cooking by commenting very briefly on one of each instrument's challenges. In the meantime, you can learn from what you have read about the violinist's head. Simply acquaint yourself with your structure and begin to analyze your misuse and correct it. This requires thinking like any other thinking; only its application is different.

VIOLA:

Since violists are generally matured violinists they bring to the viola the assets and liabilities they had as violinists. The matter of the larger size is of great concern to some and of no concern whatsoever to others. The difference is in the violist's ability to "think joints." There are four large arm joints with considerable mobility with which to accommodate the greater size. A truly tiny adjustment at each joint will make the change in either direction, from the violin to the viola or from the viola to the violin. In the fingers the same is true. The adjustments at the joints are tiny and it is those adjustments that the person who goes easily from one instrument to the other is sensing.

CELLO:

Width and length in the back are essential for cello and bass. Cellists who do not include the whole lower back in their maps, who try to play with movement from the waist up, or who are rocked too far back on their sit bones will not play easily. Cellists should look for the just right relationship of the pelvis to the chair and then, but not before, bring the instrument to them, being careful that they do not rock backward in retreat from it as it approaches, a strange habit among cellists. A cellist who approaches the cello slightly as it is brought into playing position will do fine. The contact between the player and the instrument should be fluid, not fixed. The stability for the cello is at the floor. Teachers can invite a student to move the cello all around in every direction on the endpin to see how stable and secure it is. Then the student should move all over the chair on her rockers. I call the rockers at the bottom of the pelvis the cellist's endpins. The cellist's endpins offer stability and mobility, as does the cello's endpin. What could be better? Cellists who trust the cello's stability at the floor will not overdo elsewhere by gripping at the knees or driving the cello into the chest. Cellists who have a fluid relationship with the cello at the chest and knees are always those who also comprehend their own stability at the sit bones and who move and lengthen the whole torso.

DOUBLE BASS:

Bass players needn't bend their spines. If they are free players they can get all over the bass without a great deal of spinal movement. Some tell me they choose to play without spinal movement because of the confines of the pit or the stage of the orchestra hall, or because the section leader doesn't like them to. On the other hand, the spine is a wonderful thing. Spinal movement is very efficient for coming up the fingerboard. I would certainly use spinal movement if I were a bass player, if only for the drama. The vital thing is that the head lead the movement so that the spine can lengthen. It may be failure to lead with the head that has given spinal movement a bad reputation among some players. Of course, if you fail to lead with your head, you will get a spinal shortening that will tighten your arms and worse.

Guitar:

Guitar players are the all-time spine curlers among string players. They don't all do it, but most do, and I love to watch it as much as any guitar fan. Guitar players fear that Alexander teachers will want them to uncurl, so some innate suspiciousness surfaces. Guitar players, hear this: hours and hours of curling over a guitar will not hurt you if you do it right. It will make you miserable if you do it wrong. Lead with your head, lengthen your whole spine so that your back can continually renew its lengthening and widening, stay fluid, and you'll be fine. Alexander teachers don't want to take your curl away, just your scrunch. Besides, scrunching messes up your fingers. Your arms get tired and your fingers won't do what you want them to. So, avoid scrunching, cling to lengthening and freeing as you curl, and the world is yours.

Electric Bass:

After all the fantasies I've heard about how heavy violins and violas are it was a relief to come across a truly heavy instrument. An electric bass is heavy by anybody's standards. Fortunately, human bodies are equipped to handle heavy things. Particularly they are equipped in the location where electric bass players like to sling their instruments, over their shoulders. Some bass players handle the weight comfortably week after week over a long career and others succumb to pain and numbness. Why? If a player's neck is tight so that his head is pulled forward there are three consequences that are ruinous for bass players—the pulling together of the shoulder blades, the curling forward of the upper torso in front, and the pulling down of the collarbone (plus the weight of the bass) onto the big nerves that go between the collarbone and the top rib, the pressure on which numbs the arms. Sensation returns and pain is alleviated when we reverse those conditions so that hurting bass players do what comfortable bass players have always done: balance the head, widen the back so that the shoulder blades move around toward the sides of the ribs where they belong (happily, toward the instrument), unscrunch the chest so that the pressure is taken off the nerves. Then the V formed by the collarbone and shoulder blade supports the weight of the instrument in the same way a good backpacker supports a backpack, except for its being on one side and not two.

PIANO:

Pianists are the musicians who suffer most from failing to understand the rotation of the forearm. Since they trill at the elbow joint and use it in many other ways as well it eventually gives out if it is misused. If you're a pianist, read the section of the mapping chapter dealing with the rotation of the forearm again to be SURE you understand it. Then move on to understanding the rotation of the joint of the upper arm and the shoulder blade and the rotation of the shoulder blades forward on the ribs. This latter rotation is often used effectively by free pianists in musical passages requiring great power. If you have those rotations and your primary control, you will never be tempted to have fantasies about weight.

HORN:

Should a horn player hold the instrument up or rest it on a thigh? It depends. first on what you like, and second on your build. Some short torso-ed players must rest the instrument. There isn't room not to. Some tall players can't rest the instrument without curling in a way that makes watching the conductor difficult. The decision should be made according to your structure and preference, not your teacher's.

BASSOON:

Should the bassoonist use one of the mechanical supports for the instrument now available in astonishing variety? Yes, of course, if it helps. But it won't help much if the bassoonist is pulling down. The fact is, bassoonists without downward pull rarely seek out such devices. My advice is, liberate your body's support for playing and get all the mechanical help you can get. Why not?

CLARINET:

The clarinet presents the special issue of weight on the thumb. Some clarinetists hold the instrument hours a day for a lifetime without ever thinking that it is unnatural or taxing to do so. Others are uncomfortable or exhausted by supporting the instrument and think of almost nothing else. The difference is the usual one. The difference is not in what they are doing—they are all supporting a clarinet on their thumbs—but in how they are doing it. The players who support the instrument easily have three advantages over their uncomfortable friends, and all three advantages must be in place. The first is the correct mapping of the thumb (three bony segments, not two), the second is the correct mapping of the rotation of the lower arm (no instrument can be supported on a radius), and the third is, you guessed it, the absence of downward pull. Downward pull tenses the arms in proportion to the tensing of the torso, and tensed muscles do a poor job of bearing weight. I invite clarinetists to try an experiment, which is to leave the instrument in the case and play an imaginary clarinet for a while, leaving all the usual tensing in place, supporting the imaginary clarinet in the same way they support the clarinet that is in the case. The clarinetist usually experiences the same discomfort and fatigue playing the imaginary clarinet as the real one, proving that it is not the weight of the clarinet, but the habits of the clarinetist, that are the problem.

TRUMPET, TROMBONE AND TUBA:

Everything in the breathing chapter applies to you. Sheer destructive fantasy about breathing plagues brass players as it does singers and other wind players.

FLUTE:

Sometimes flute players find they have more tension on one side of their necks than on the other because of the way they turn their heads. This is directly related to misuse and it results eventually in a torquing of the jaw at its joints with the skull. When it occurs it gives the player strange sensations, "I can open one side of my throat more than the other," or "I can't breathe through one nostril." When the neck is uniformly freed, the jaw tends to come back home.

OBOE:

Double reed players worry about the necessity for pressure against the reed. I don't know how that pressure is created. That is a technical issue which I leave up to the double reed teachers, though I suspect that it's a little like wiggling your ears. It's not very teachable. Probably you have to fool around until you figure it out internally. What I am absolutely certain of is this: whatever it takes to secure that pressure is not visible and it is not external. Free, efficient oboe players do not do anything different with the muscles on the surface of their bodies than the free flute players and clarinetists sitting next to them. The pressure is secured internally, where the air actually is. When double reed players get rid of the tensing on the surface they are usually able to figure out what they have to do inside, and they can't believe how easy it is, compared to what they were doing.

Wind players have a challenge with their fingers that brass players know nothing about, and I think that wind teachers need to address this directly with their students, likewise Alexander teachers. The work it takes to depress the valves on a brass instrument is the same valve to valve. Not true of wind instruments. Some fingers cover holes, so all the work that is needed is whatever it takes to cover the hole reliably. Some fingers depress keys that can be depressed by the weight of the finger alone, so no work whatsoever is required, only the delivery of the weight of the finger onto the key. Other fingers will rest on the key without depressing it. Work is required, very little, but some. The wind player's challenge is to discover just how much work is involved in each instance, because overwork ties up the whole hand. I suggest that wind players leave their instruments out on a table or sit with them in your laps as you watch television or chat with friends. Let your fingers play with the keys, using an unaccustomed finger most of the time. The fingers will gradually teach themselves just what is required at each key. Muscles are great learners.

PERCUSSION:

The freest players on most concert stages—rock concerts, jazz concerts, symphony concerts, country concerts, concert band—are the percussion players. Wonder why? Maybe it's all the movement they do? Maybe it's some mystique? Maybe it's because drums sound so terrible played tensely? Maybe it's because there's a self-conscious element of dance in drumming? Maybe it's because we have unconscious expectations about how drummers should look—we expect them to look free?

When percussionists are in trouble it is usually because they are compromising the mechanical integrity of weight delivery onto the floor. This is compounded if they don't have hip joints mapped properly, making it uncomfortable simply to move their feet to go to one end of a marimba or the other. Percussionists are also prone to wrist and elbow problems, which almost always clear up with a return to proper use.

Appendix III. If You're a Singer

Many singers struggle in intense frustration against the effect of downward pull on their bodies. They know they are not getting the air they ought to have, and they don't know why. They know they are not getting the resonance they ought to have, and they don't know why. They know articulation and support should be easier than they are. They also know that most remedies suggested to them don't work, and they don't know why.

Singers' teachers are as frustrated as the students. Over and over again I hear, "I don't know what I'm going to do with Susie. Nothing I tell her works. She can't do anything I ask her to, and yet she's an earnest person and she really wants to sing. I think there's a voice in there somewhere." The teachers are frustrated because for all they know, much of it sophisticated, they don't know how to recognize downward pull or alleviate it. They know their students are tense but they don't know that the tension comes in a whole-body pattern or that the pattern has an organization and an ultimate source. They don't know tension in the throat is inevitable when there is tension in the neck or that tension in the torso is inevitable when there is tension in the neck, and they don't comprehend the patterned tension that exerts a tyranny over the singing structures of the body so powerful that nothing can counter it. The sad fact is: *to the extent* that Susie is pulled down Susie will be limited in her singing. The only real hope for Susie is the alleviation of downward pull.

Karl Resnik told me that it wasn't until he became acquainted with the insights of F. M. Alexander that he figured out why some students could learn what he taught and others could not. It was a question he had asked himself again and again. He would say the same things to the student at 10 AM that he had just successfully taught to the student at 9 AM, but the 10 AM student couldn't begin to do what Karl asked, or could do some things and not others, or could do something for a moment and would then go right back to the old way. When Karl understood that a student who is not pulled down and who has a correct map can easily follow an instruction to, for instance, drop the jaw, or lift the soft palate, or bring the tongue slightly forward, and that a student who is pulled down will find two of these things impossible and the other difficult, he had the answer to his question.

When I talk to groups of singing teachers I carry with me a large anatomical chart showing the muscles of the body as seen from front and back. The muscles are beautiful, really, and impressively massive and complex. I remind the teachers as they look at the chart that no muscle visible in either picture except the lips has anything to do with singing. The charts provide a dramatic reminder that singing is a profoundly interior activity. Think about it. Interior to the massive cylinder of movement muscle that lies under our skins reside the singing structures—the resonating spaces and the shaping muscles, the vocal chords, the lungs, the diaphragm, and the support musculature of the lower torso. All wrapped up like a baby in a blanket, and a delicate baby it is. The delicate baby, which should be protected and warmed by the blanket, is, in downward pull, nearly squeezed to death by it. The baby can't breathe or move. The baby is miserable, and nothing will help except loosening the blanket.

The singers who do musical theatre need the blanket free as much as they need the baby free, for the muscles that contract in the pattern of tension we call downward pull are the muscles that do the dramatic part of singing, the acting and the dancing, the gesturing and the bowing. Singers are as limited dramatically by downward pull as they are limited vocally. When singers improve vocally using the Technique they also improve in overall expressiveness. Please, if you do musical theatre, or if you want to improve the expressive effectiveness of your recitals, read the chapter on acting. Everything said there applies to you.

Whom do you believe?

Nothing could be more confusing than the advice given to singers by other singers. The singing texts contain the most appalling contradictions. Whom do you believe? What do you do? Well, you have to get out the hardy little boat of your intelligence and sail the choppy sea of contradiction until you pull up onto a beach of understanding. That's what Alexander did, and he healed his voice. You must return again and again to the simple truth of your structure. If you read or hear an instruction that is contrary to your structure, scrap it. It can't work.

Unless it's an image? Teachers say to me, "Well, when I tell students to take air into their bellies, I don't really mean that. I do really know that if air goes in their bellies, they die. But I mean they should feel like they have air in their bellies. They should use the image of having air in their bellies." And, of course, sometimes the image actually liberates some of the power of the support stuff in the belly. I say sometimes, because it will work if the student isn't pulled down but it hasn't a prayer if she is. Or, the student may have a little more support but no more understanding and she has the added burden of using her imagination about her body rather than about the text and the character.

If you are the student of such a teacher, ask yourself just exactly what your teacher means in structural terms. Then when your teacher says, "Fill your belly!" you can rapidly translate, "Oh, yeah, by that he means that I should allow the movement of inhalation to travel throughout my whole torso, that I should stay kinesthetically awake and released in the whole of me, and that on the exhalation I should lengthen in order to engage the support of my primary control, the support muscles of my pelvic cavity and my pelvic floor. Okay. Here goes." Your teacher will say, "Finally you're getting what I've been saying to you."

If you read a book like Jerome Hines' *Great Singers on Great Singing* you will read as much contradiction as it is possible for one book to sustain, and as much nonsense. On only one point is there agreement, the necessity for freedom from tension. My theory is that singers who go to the top of the profession have the outrageous good fortune of having never lost their primary control. They talk about singing out of their own experience of it, which tends to focus on the structure of the feeling rather than the movement, like the feeling of the "fire in the belly" or the buzzing of the skull. These people have that luxury, because they are free enough to actually support from their bellies and create bone resonance in the head. But the difficulty is that no pulled-down person will ever feel either thing until he's free, and, in the meantime, if he tries to create in himself the same feelings the free singer has described his only recourse is imagination or more tension, in which case he has just gone to a fine restaurant and eaten the menu and menus taste yucky.

So, if you are pulled down and desperate to sing and willing to make the journey in your little boat, you must, as I see it, become intimately acquainted with your own body, recover your primary control, and then watch singers you admire like a hawk for what they actually do, for you will learn very little from what they say they do or what they advise you to do. Go to concerts and watch. Get video tapes and watch. Imitate everything you see. Analyze it minutely. Boxers have been doing that for years. Why not you? The funny thing is, those singers in Hines's book *do* the same things, they just name them differently. Get as free as they are and you'll have the luxury of naming any old way you like, too.

Beret Arcaya, an Alexander teacher who is herself a singer, wrote an article for our professional journal, *NASTAT News*, about singing, in which she recommended a book which I, too, recommend. It is *Hints on Singing* by Manuel Garcia, translated from the French, edited, expanded, and arranged by Hermann Klein, who describes it as "the most concise and compact treatise on the Art of Singing yet given to the world." He goes on, "the contents of this volume consist of a great deal more than mere 'hints.' Apart from being his last word on the subject, they embody all the profound knowledge, the penetrating observation, the rich experience, the logical deductions and conclusions of three-quarters of a century of active devotion to the study and practice of vocal science." Garcia was the teacher of Jenny Lind, and his book is available from the Joseph Patelson Music House, 160 West 56th Street, New York, NY 10019.

Appendix IV. If You're a Dancer

Imagine yourself at a party. A stranger walks up to you and inquires, "Are you a dancer?" "Yes," you reply, "how did you know?" If the stranger says, "It's your aura of extraordinary kindness," or, "There are toe shoes sticking out of your bag," you're okay. If the stranger says, "I dunno, it's something about the way you stand," be worried. The stranger means, "Your neck is awfully straight, your sternum is hoisted, your shoulders are dropped down and back, there's an unusual over-arching of your back, you carry your tailbone real low, your thighs are torqued out, and your ankles look like they're trying to get away from each other."

Fact is, there is a pattern of tension shared by many dancers in our time that is easily parodied and would be endearing if it didn't cause so much plain old misery. It not only renders dancers susceptible to injury but it also impairs performance, because not much that is fresh or engaging can emerge out of bodies in a ubiquitous dancerly grip. Choreographers invent around the grip, but from the audience the grip is the overwhelming impression. Invention is lost and audiences are bored.

Dancers who use Alexander can liberate their bodies from both classic downward pull, which the grip is often superimposed on, and from the Grip, allowing the dancers' uniqueness to emerge and extending technical capacity.

That is, if it's real Alexander, the liberating kind. Sometimes one sees a dancer who has layered a third "Alexander habit" over the other two habits, yet another stiffness, yet another "rightness." This is misery on misery and takes a deal of sorting out. The basic questions one must ask assume a towering significance: Is it easier? Is it freer? Is it better balanced? Is it more supported? Is it lighter? Is it more comfortable? Does it promote full energy? full expression of emotion? full range of motion? full technical mastery? If not, it ain't it. Dancer, you must wend your way down through the layers of conditioned rightness like some goddess looking for her lost child in the circles of hell until you retrieve your primary control and the artistry that accrues to it. Nothing is more demanding of your sensibility and clarity. Nothing is more worthy.

Every dancer should be acquainted from the beginning with the spine and its laws. There should be pictures of spines and full-size skeletons in every dance studio and teachers of dance should refer the students constantly to their experience of their spines. Spines organize vertebrate movement. Every great dancer of every sort understands that, and you can watch that understanding in operation. It's easy to see it once you know how to look for it. In all the dancers' movement the primary movement is the lengthening and freeing of the spine and everything else that is happening is organized by that primary movement and is dependent on it for its integrity. The limbs have an integrated *and* autonomous organization *and* freedom when the primary movement is primary that disintegrates as soon as the primary movement fails.

Unless you are one of the fortunates in this world who never interfered with her primary control and whose body map is accurate and available and whose kinesthesia is refined and reliable you will need to study the spine and weed out all illusions about it in your thinking. The truth about the spine is probably far friendlier than your fantasies about it, so discovering the truth should be enjoyable and encouraging. Besides noticing its convincing size and its reassuring centrality in your torso and its lovely curves to help it with the impact of jumping, notice also and particularly its jointedness. The spine is a series of twenty-four joints. You must be like the scientists here. Scientists have two ways of looking at tiny particles, depending on their purpose. Sometimes scientists look at particles as waves, which they are, because that is the only way to look that satisfies the scientists' purpose, and sometimes scientists look at particles as things, which they are, because that is the only way that satisfies another purpose. You will think of the spine as many nicely cushioned bones beautifully designed to deliver weight and support movement when your purpose is mechanical advantage, but you will look at the spine as the spaces between the bones when your purpose is movement and reflex support.

There are many millions of years of evolution behind the dancer's leading with her head, even pre-vertebrate evolution. Bill Conable once gave an introductory lecture about the Alexander Technique in which he said, "How can you tell which is the front end of a worm, anyway?" Dancers should learn to watch every sort of creature with the central dynamic of the body in mind, the lengthening-sequencing at the core. When the head is leading and the spine following, all movement is organized and supported by the core lengthening, and it is that organization and support that gives movement its breathtaking beauty and integrity.

Dancers are often confused when they hear this dynamic first spoken of, and the confusion has two sources, first the importance accorded the Center in the pelvis. This confusion is allayed when a dancer actually takes Alexander lessons because the dancer quickly learns that the Alexander teacher appreciates and admires the pelvis at least as much as the dancer does. Indeed, the teacher wants to help the dancer to a poise of the head and a lengthening of the spine that will liberate the pelvis, because the pelvis, like many other structures, loses mobility in proportion to the imposition of downward pull and regains mobility in proportion to a reduction of downward pull. When downward pull is reduced to the point where the spine can actually consistently lengthen in movement, then the dancer can regain full pelvic mobility, and not before. We free the neck and spine in order to free the pelvis and the limbs. Full pelvic mobility is secured by a lengthening spine which allows for an engagement and lengthening of the deep pelvic musculature. As the lower lower back widens in movement rather than narrowing (as it does in the Grip) and the pelvic floor releases in movement rather than hiking up (as it does in the Grip) then the hip joints can free and the legs come out of the torquing that is characteristic of both downward pull and the Grip.

The second source of confusion is the matter of initiation. Dancers will ask, "How can I initiate the movement from the head when I have been told to initiate it at the shoulder or the hip?" This initiation matter is simple once you understand it, so bear with me please while I try to explain.

Initiation is defined this way: a part of the body moves first, with resulting movement in other parts of the body. A dancer whose arm is extended to the side can initiate movement at his fingertips and a ripple of resulting movement can flow through his body to the tips of his toes and through to his other hand, simultaneously bringing the head toward the initiating fingertips. It's a beautiful thing to watch. It is this initiation that Laban notation records and that choreographers first imagine and then teach and that audiences watch with satisfaction. Here's the point. The integrity of that choreographed movement depends on another initiation, the initiation of the spinal core of the movement at the head.

As the dancer initiates with his fingertips and the rest of his body responds his spine will either lengthen or shorten. Those are the two things spines do in movement. If his spine shortens he will not experience the beautiful flowing through the body that the initiation ought to involve because he will be too tense. If, on the other hand, his spine lengthens as he initiates from his fingertips the resulting movement in his body will be everything he desires because it will be organized and supported by the his anti-gravity reflexes in all their glory. The spinal lengthening depends on his neck being free enough to allow his head to lead the spinal movement that provides the core of the choreographed movement.

So two initiations are occurring at once, one notated and taught, the other assumed. The fingertips are initiating the choreographed movement and the head is initiating the spinal movement that supports and organizes the choreographed movement.

The spinal movement is constantly re-initiated, constantly renewed, in beautiful dancing. The success of all other initiations in the body depends on the presence of the initiation of the primary movement of the spine. Lucy Venable once called it a pre-initiation. It is the condition for the magic in dance.

Appendix V. If You're an Actor

In the my theatre movement class at the Cincinnati Conservatory I taught the young actors the movement capabilities I observe in fine acting. I told the students in the first class that I would write them a check for $100 if they would bring me a tape of a fine performance in which the actor did not exhibit the following qualities:

- inclusive awareness

- an accurate body map

- adherence to Alexander's principles

- complete or nearly complete range of motion in all the joints

- an understanding that speech and singing are movement

- a kinesthetic imagination

I didn't lose any money on this offer. I reminded the students again and again that it is the actors with those qualities who win auditions. In many instances the actor is simply exhibiting qualities he or she by some mercy never lost. When these qualities are lost, they can be recovered, but only by application and intention. The information necessary to recover all of these qualities with the help of a good teacher is provided in this book, except for the last, kinesthetic imagination. Most actors can use already existing training exercises and their own life experience to cultivate a kinesthetic imagination as soon as they understand what it is.

Kinesthetic imagination is movement imagined *as movement*, not visualized. It is the actor internally *feeling* the character's movement rather than internally seeing it, which makes all the difference in the quality and complexity of the resulting movement. The actor who imagines a movement kinesthetically and then does it looks alive in the doing. The actor who imagines a movement visually and then does it looks wooden or disembodied and the movement rarely has the complexity to be interesting. Often it is strangely stereotyped.

Some actors become adept at translating from their visual imaginations to their kinesthetic, often at the last minute in the preparation of a role, so the director is desperate about what's on stage at the dress rehearsal and breathes a sigh of relief at the performance because the movement on the stage comes alive finally. Translating from one sensory mode into another is better than not translating but it is an unnecessary burden on the actor. If the actor conceives of movement from the very beginning with the kinesthetic imagination, if the actor cultivates a movement imagination that is lively and varied, if the actor can amuse herself in that mode with an engaged attention, then we see a wonderful result, an actor at home in movement. This can be learned, and then it can be cultivated. Student actors should leave the visual imagination to the scene designers and the costume people and to learn to feel movement in its own terms.

A bonus here is that an actor with a developed movement imagination can use it to good effect in enhancing primary control. One actor who took a workshop unobtrusively imitated the movement out of downward pull as he observed it in the other participants. He never needed to be guided because he moved up beautifully in response to what he saw.

The Matter of the Mask

I was puzzled by a certain facial immobility in the actors in my movement class, the very persons on earth who need mobile faces. I asked the students about it. "How do you think about your face?" I asked. "I do this with the mask, or that," they replied. I inquired into what a facial mask is, how it works. I got vague answers that I couldn't understand. Then I said, "Just describe a face. What's it made of?" The students all named skin, some of them named bone, only a couple had any sense of there being muscle between the two. I passed out pictures of the facial muscles. I said I thought mask was a lousy metaphor for a face. A mask is immobile, and in contrast the muscles of the face move it all over the place. The students played with the muscles of their faces and got back some mobility. I encouraged them to learn to wiggle their ears and to wiggle their scalps back and forth over their skulls. I was surprised to find that this helped them free their necks as well. It seems that when they froze their faces into a mask they also froze their necks.

One lesson in the matter of the mask—listen to the language you use about your body. Especially examine the metaphors, which so often have unfortunate consequences in movement. Inquire of yourself.

Appendix VI: Finding Good Books About the Alexander Technique

John Coffin

The Alexander Technique does not fit neatly into the categories offered by most publishers. Bookstores and libraries may carry several titles on the Technique, only to scatter them on their shelves under such headings as Drama, Health, Psychology, Philosophy, Meditation, Fitness, Self-Help, 'New-Age,' etc. Over the years, a trickle of books have been produced in which the Technique has been misrepresented in order to fit these categories. Two types in particular have appeared: books which purport to teach the Technique on a do-it-yourself basis; and books in which the Technique has been entangled with pop-psychology, health fads, or cults. These books have harmed the growth and reputation of the Alexander Technique. Readers of how-to books are either led to believe that the Alexander Technique consists of a few trivial exercises or visualizations, or are so frustrated by their lack of progress that they feel the Technique to be impractical or too arduous to be realistically considered. Faddish books repel the serious inquirer, and may leave many readers feeling that having had a massage or purchased a crystal, they already know all about the Alexander Technique.

Some fine books about the Technique do contain material for self instruction; these passages are usually intended for people who have already had lessons (Like John Gray's *Your Guide to the Alexander Technique*), or draw from other disciplines (e.g. Deborah Caplan's physical therapy-based exercises for back-pain sufferers in *Back Trouble*). Other writers have contributed very good articles on the Technique to alternative health collections or guides, for whose content the publishers disclaim any responsibility, usually in small print. A clear presentation of the Technique suffers by being included with articles promoting dubious therapies. Other books are burdened by jacket blurbs which falsely assign them to these categories.

Sources for Books

If your bookstore or library does not have the titles below, it would be a great service if you would request that they stock some of them, this would make matters easier for subsequent inquirers who might be too shy to ask. As it would be unreasonable to expect most stores to carry more than a few titles, here are some addresses for a wider selection:

AmSTAT Books
P.O. Box 517
Urbana, IL 61801
USA
1-800-473-0620
www.alexandertech.org

AmSTAT books offer full access to Alexander Technique materials currently in print.

STAT Books
20 London House
266 Fulham Road
London, SW10 9EL
England

A staff of volunteers from the Society of Teachers of the Alexander Technique will fill orders for a impressive list of books, pamphlets and videos.

Recommended Books

Note: This list is meant to be a brief guide. I give my full recommendation to the titles I have included. Exclusion from this list should not be considered a negative comment on the worth of any book. There are books on the Technique which I would condemn, but it is not my intention to do so here.

Basic Introductions

Stevens, Chris. *Alexander Technique*. Illustrated by Shaun Williams. London: Macdonald and Co., 1987. This clear, accessible, 111-page book answers many of the prospective student's most common questions, *e.g.*: What is the Alexander technique? For what reasons do people take lessons? How do I find a teacher? etc. Further, the book gives a chapter to a review of the experimental work confirming the physiological soundness of the Technique and a short list of relevant books and articles.

Gelb, Michael. *Body Learning: An introduction to the Alexander Technique*. London: Aurum Press, 1981; revised edition 1994. Beautifully illustrated with carefully selected photographs. In three parts, Gelb gives: first, a brief account of Alexander's discovery, second, a series of short chapters exploring basic principles of the Technique (the meat of the book), and last; some notes on using the Technique in various situations and on the application of the Technique in the education of children. The new edition adds a fourth section which answers practical questions about finding teachers, what lessons are like, etc. The book also has a very fine bibliography.

Taken together, these two volumes should be of tremendous help to the prospective or beginning student. If your local library or bookstore doesn't carry any books on the Technique, recommend these titles.

The Next Step

Jones, Frank Pierce. *Body Awareness in Action*. New York: Schocken Books, 1976, 1979. To date, the richest and most informative book on the Technique. Jones reviews the history of the Technique, summarizes Alexander's books, gives an account of his own experiences as student, trainee and teacher, and gives a short presentation of the contents of his 31 published experimental papers. Some beginners may find this book a little rich for their blood, but this is the one to take to that desert island; the superb bibliography alone is worth the price of the book. Required reading for serious students and teachers. The State University of New York Press will reissue *Body Awareness* and a volume of collected papers of Frank Pierce Jones within the next year; both volumes will be available from NASTAT Books.

These first three titles constitute a core of information that would be hard to improve upon.

More Technical
(But not necessarily less readable)

Dart, Raymond A. *Skill and Poise*. N.p, n.d. R.A. Dart, the anatomist and paleo-anthropologist (the first to identify hominid fossils in Africa, the namer of Australo-pithecus) studied the Technique briefly in 1943. When the only Alexander teacher in South Africa returned to England, Dart combined what he had learned of the Technique with his enormous knowledge of human anatomy and phylogeny to develop a self-exploratory system now known as the Dart Procedures, still taught and practiced by many Alexander teachers. This collection of papers includes: Dart's three major works on human posture, coordination, and the Alexander Technique; an illustrated presentation of the Procedures by Alexander Murray, and a selection of papers filling out Dart's ideas.

Garlick, David. *The Lost Sixth Sense: a medical scientists looks at the Alexander Technique*. University of New South Wales School of Physiology and Pharmacology, 1990. Really a large pamphlet. Garlick, a professor of physiology, presents his understanding of the Technique and explains much of what is now known of the underlying mechanisms in layman's terms, accompanied by helpful drawings. A fine resource for students and teachers. It is wonderful to see a well-written book by a student of the Technique. Marred by the lack of references or a bibliography.

Gorman, David. *The Body Movable*. 3 vols. Guelph, Ontario: Ampersand Printing Co., 1981. Gorman, an Alexander teacher and a fine illustrator, has assembled an exhaustively thorough study of the anatomy of movement.

Not Directly about the Technique
(but very helpful)

Kapit, Wynn, and Lawrence M. Elson. *The Anatomy Coloring Book*. New York: Harper Collins Publishers, 1977; 2nd edition, revised and expanded, 1993. Widely available and easy to use, this standard book is a wonderful reference, even if you haven't colored all the plates.

Tobias, Phillip V. *Man, the tottering biped. The evolution of his posture, poise and skill*. University of New South Wales, 1982. This, the opening address of Dr. Garlick's 1981 symposium: "Proprioception, Posture and Emotion" was given by Tobias in place of the absent Raymond Dart. Although Tobias is not a student of the Technique and only refers to the Alexander Technique in passing, this short, accessible book will reward any interested reader. With its view of the evolutionary development, comparative anatomy, and startling potential of our unique relationship to gravity, this will open the eyes of anyone who feels or has been told that human bipedalism is some sort of evolutionary mistake.

Also

Caplan, Deborah. *Back Trouble: A New Approach to Prevention and Recovery*. Gainesville, Florida: Triad Publishing Company, 1987. A useful 'two-fer.' Caplan is both an Alexander teacher and a physical therapist. She begins with a clear presentation of the technique as she teaches it, with a focus on back pain. The later parts of the book are full of advice and exercises only partly connected to the Alexander Technique as such.

Alexander's Books

These are still the primary source of information on the Technique. Much has been said and written against these books. They are said to be "too difficult...badly written...dated," or "politically incorrect." The more I read these books, the feebler the objections seem. Alexander was not by any standard a fluent or elegant writer, but he wrote these books with enormous care, and they hold the most complete expression of the Technique. Recent criticisms, from readers new to the books and unacquainted with their period, make much of the presence of the language, current at that time, of social or racial ranking, and the eugenics movement. While Alexander was as interested in the development of human potential as the eugenicists were, he was not a biological determinist at all. In *Man's Supreme Inheritance* he wrote: "no reasoning person can doubt...that in the vast majority of cases at least, the influence of heredity can be practically eradicated."

Man's Supreme Inheritance (1910) and *Conscious Control* (1912). These two early works have been re-issued in one volume by Centerline Press. Brief and readable, they suffer from having been rushed to print to forestall plagiarists. Included as an appendix is an even earlier pamphlet, "Re-education of the Kinesthetic Systems."

Man's Supreme Inheritance (1918). The most popular of Alexander's books during his lifetime, combining and greatly expanding the material in the first two books. This represents a real attempt to represent the work completely in print. Modern readers will have to squirm through some overconfident claims, archaic medical folklore, and Alexander's naive acceptance of contemporary American anthropological pseudo-science. Not in print since the late 1950's, this book is worth finding. Held in many university libraries.

Constructive Conscious Control of the Individual (1923). Alexander considered this to be a second volume to *Man's Supreme Inheritance*, and his best book. The longest of the books, this again represents an attempt at a full representation of the Technique. Lacks index.

The Use of the Self (1932). Since Alexander's death, this book has grown in reputation and is now generally considered the most accessible and practical of the books. Alexander gives a thorough account of his original experiments, and examples of the application of the technique to students.

The Universal Constant in Living (1941). A sort of footnote to the previous books. The Universal Constant jumps around from chapter to chapter and lacks a unifying story line, but Alexander never wrote more effectively than in this book. Much material from the earlier works is restated with beautiful clarity. The introduction by the American anatomist/neurologist George Ellet Coghill is a must-read for serious students.

Authorised Summaries of F. M. Alexander's Four Books. Edited by Ron Brown.
    Reuter's correspondent Ronald Brown wrote these summaries in the late
    1940's as part of an unfinished larger project. Alexander reviewed and
    approved these summaries, initialing them page by page. Rediscovered in
    the 1980's and published by STAT Books, this volume is a tremendous
    boon to contemporary students; the clean, compressed presentation
    should enable any reader to grasp the core arguments of Alexander's
    writing.

Alexander Technique: The Essential Writings of F. Matthias Alexander. Edited by
    Edward Maisel. (originally issued in 1969 as *The Resurrection of the Body*).
    A collection of extracts from Alexander's books, with a long introduction by Maisel and
    the introductory essays of John Dewey and Coghill. Marred by Maisel's oddly slanted
    introduction: he insists the Technique can be learned on a how-to basis and derisively
    dismisses any hint that the Technique might have educational or philosophical signifi-
    cance.

Some Worthwhile Articles

Over the years, a number of articles on the technique have appeared which
rise far above the level of popular endorsements or "therapy smorgasbords."
Wilfred Barlow collected many of them in his book, *More Talk of Alexander*,
now unfortunately out of print. A university library should have at least some
of the following articles; if they do not, or you have no access to a university,
your public library's interlibrary loan service should be able to get some of
them for you.

Robinson, James Harvey. "The Philosopher's Stone." *Atlantic Monthly* (Febru-
    ary 1918): 474-81. The great Columbia professor of history introduced Alexander's
    teaching, and his first book, to the American public with this article. Still one of the best
    introductions to the Technique.

Macdonald, Peter. "Instinct and Functioning in Health and Disease." *British
    Medical Journal* 2 (December 1926): 1221-23. In his presidential address to the
    Yorkshire branch of the British Medical Association, Dr. Macdonald gives a clear
    presentation of the Technique from the viewpoint of an informed student.

Barlow, Wilfred. "An Investigation Into Kinaesthesia." *Medical Press and
    Circular* 215 (1946): 60. During the War, Dr. Barlow performed this elegant explora-
    tion of "downward pull" in officer cadets. Alexander assisted in the writing of this paper.

———————————"Postural Homeostasis." *Annals of Physical Medicine* 1 (July
    1952): 77-89. In the early 1950s, Barlow supervised photographic studies on students
    in performing arts schools in London, comparing the results of Alexander instruction
    with postural exercises. All the schools involved adopted the Technique as a result of
    these studies. This paper includes the largest selection of the before and after photo-
    graphs of students which Barlow used in his later papers and books.

—————————"Psychosomatic Problems in Postural Re-education." *The Lancet* (September 2, 1955): 659 ff. A presentation of the Technique for doctors.

Jones, Frank Pierce. "Method for Changing Stereotyped Response Patterns by the Inhibition of Certain Postural Sets." *Psychological Review* 72 (1965): 196-214. A beautiful presentation, summarizing Jones's experiments up to 1965. Jones does not seek to prove the Technique by before and after demonstrations, which can seldom effectively demonstrate a link between cause and effect. He is instead concerned with exploring the measurable influence of changes in the head-neck relation on movement patterns. The results are fascinating; this paper is a must for those seriously interested in the Technique.

—————————"Postural Set and Overt Movement: a Force-platform Analysis." *Perceptual and Motor Skills* 30 (1970): 699-702.

—————————"Voice Production as a Function of Head Balance in Singers." *Journal of Psychology* 82 (1972): 209-215. Two later papers of Jones in which newer techniques are used.

Austin, John; and Ausubel, Pearl. "Enhanced Respiratory Muscular Function in Normal Adults after Lessons in Proprioceptive Musculoskeletal Education without Exercises." *Chest*, 102 (August 2, 1992): pp. 486-490. The Technique is well presented in this recent study, the improvements in breathing which have been subjectively reported for a century are demonstrated in concrete form.

John Coffin, a member of the North American Society of Teachers of the Alexander Technique, and the National Council Against Health Fraud, is a graduate of the Alexander Training Institute of San Francisco. He is currently an assistant teacher at ATISF, and sings with the San Francisco Opera Chorus.

About the Authors

Barbara Conable is a member of the North American Society for the Teachers of the Alexander Technique and Alexander Technique International. She began her study of the Technique in 1961 and has been teaching the Technique since 1975 in Columbus, Ohio, where she has an extensive private practice. With other teachers she offers two residence courses yearly, one in Virginia in July, and one in Columbus between Christmas and New Years. She is the editor of *Marjorie Barstow: Her Teaching and Training*, a book of essays about the teaching of Marjorie Barstow.

William Conable, designer and illustrator of this book and author of the chapter on the origins and theory of mapping, is Professor of Music at the Ohio State University and was for eleven years Principal Cellist of the Columbus Symphony Orchestra. He was a pupil of Marjorie Barstow and the late Frank Pierce Jones. His course in the Alexander Technique at OSU, established in 1973, was one of the first university courses in the Technique. He teaches with Barbara Conable at the residence courses mentioned above and has given workshops in both music and the Alexander Technique at universities in the US and in Europe.

About this Book

This manual is being issued in small printings and is being continually revised in order to make it increasingly useful to students and teachers. Barbara Conable would very much appreciate feedback or suggestions from readers. Feel free to write her at 4427 North Willis Blvd., Portland, OR 97203.